Contents at a Glance

Table of Contents

Part II: Focusing on Your Personal Development.. 43

Chapter 3: Weighing Academic Qualifications 45

Chapter 4: Professional Requirements: How Do You Rate? 65

Introduction

. . . .

So, you want to be a nurse? That's a great ambition and one that many people aspire to. So many people, in fact, that nursing is one of the most popular courses at UK universities. But there are many more applications than places available, and ultimately, each year many candidates are disappointed.

That's why, if you're to succeed in your nursing application, you need help and advice to plan your way forward. And that's what this book is all about – clear, practical guidance from an experienced nursing admissions tutor that helps you make your application stand out from the rest.

A nursing application can take many years to prepare, and the application and selection processes are only the first stages in your long journey to become a qualified nurse. If you're ready to take on this challenge then read on . . . and welcome to nursing.

About This Book

This book is born of my experience as both a nurse lecturer and an admissions tutor:

- ✔ **Selecting candidates:** I spend a considerable part of my working week selecting future nursing students, and over the years I have seen many thousands of ambitious and eager candidates. Some of the candidates have gone on to be highly successful nurses, such as ward managers and senior nurses. Others missed out on opportunities and never made it past the interview stage.

- ✔ **Teaching students:** A registered nurse, I spend the other part of my week teaching students at university and supporting them while in clinical practice, so I know a lot about students and how they cope with the nursing course.

These combined experiences have given me an in-depth understanding of what draws people to nursing, why some do well while others fail, and how to differentiate between the excellent, the good and the not-so-good candidate.

In this book, then, you get an insider's perspective into what it takes to succeed in an application. I lead you through the whole process of getting into nursing school, from preparing your application through to getting that all-important offer letter, showing you the different aspects that you're likely to encounter – and, crucially, how to handle them.

Conventions Used in This Book

Throughout the book I use a few conventions:

- I use *italics* for emphasis and to highlight new words or concepts.
- **Boldfaced** text indicates key words in bulleted lists or the key steps of action lists.
- `Monofont` indicates internet and email addresses. If you're reading this book on an enabled device, the web addresses are hyperlinked.
- Sidebars, the shaded grey boxes that you occasionally see, give examples to support the discussion, handy tips and background information.
- In the interests of balance, I alternate male and female pronouns between chapters.

What You're Not to Read

Whether you're completely new to nursing or have many years of nursing experience, this book offers all you need to make that all-important good impression on admissions tutors. But candidates who arrive at the decision to apply for nursing come from a wide variety of backgrounds, and so following the logical order of chapters doesn't necessarily suit your need for information. Well, that's okay, because each chapter of this book is self-contained and gives you the relevant information and advice for that particular topic. So don't feel that you need to read the entire book from start to end: if you already have a good knowledge of the subject that I explore in a chapter then just move on to the next one.

Foolish Assumptions

Having been an admissions tutor for many years and seen many candidates in that time, I have come to understand what the usual candidate is like and what draws them to nursing. With this in mind I have made a few assumptions about you, the reader.

Well, the first assumption is actually not to assume too much! Candidates come from all walks of life and I am always surprised at just how diverse the backgrounds of nursing candidates are. With this in mind there are a few things that I *don't* assume:

  ✔ That you are of a particular age or gender. Whether you're a young woman or a middle-aged man has no bearing on my consideration about you. Age and gender don't influence your suitability to nursing.

  ✔ Your cultural influences, spiritual beliefs, ethnicity or nationality. None of these make you better or worse than any other candidate and so I take no regard of these.

I've given much consideration to why you've picked up this book and where you're coming from. With this in mind I assume that:

  ✔ You want to become a nurse and have a real interest in succeeding with your application. This book gives you the advice you need to improve your chances. However, I assume that you're motivated and will put some hard work in preparing your application.

  ✔ You have some understanding of nursing. Although I explain in some detail what nursing in the UK is about, you need to have an appreciation of the basic role of the nurse.

  ✔ That you appreciate the importance of education in preparing for your application.

  ✔ You like being around people! Nursing is about people and you need to want and like to be with people. Being highly intelligent with a great academic profile doesn't necessarily make a good nurse. You must want to work alongside people to succeed with your application.

How This Book Is Organised

This book contains six parts, each of which breaks down into a number of chapters. Each part explores an important aspect of planning your application, and the chapters develop in more detail the various considerations relating to that part. Here's a summary of each part.

Part I: Getting Started with a Career in Nursing

If you're going to spend the rest of your working life as a nurse, the first step is to understand what nursing is. The nursing profession is a national institution that underpins all healthcare within the UK and it's regulated to ensure that citizens are offered top-quality care. This part helps explain how nursing has developed into the profession it is today, and it offers you insight into the different types of nursing and the opportunities available to you after you qualify.

Part II: Focusing on Your Personal Development

Nursing attracts people from all walks of life and this diversity is one of its strengths. Identifying what qualities and experiences you have that support your application can make you a strong candidate. But equally, you need to identify which areas you need to develop. This part explores what it takes to be a nurse – from qualifications and care experience through to meeting professional requirements and demonstrating the necessary skills and qualities.

Part III: Preparing to Apply

Higher education is a whole new world, and with so many universities and courses on offer, the task of making suitable choices can be daunting. In this section I explain how university nursing programmes work, to help you select the right course. I give you a helping hand in exploring universities to see which best suit your requirements and offer some helpful tips for attending open days. I round off with a look at financial affairs – so you can be sure you can afford to study.

Part IV: Perfecting Your Application

After all your preparation, you don't want a poor application to let you down. The Universities and Colleges Admissions Service (UCAS) process can appear complicated and difficult to navigate should you not be aware how it works. This part explains in detail how the UCAS application process works and the tasks you need to carry out. I give specific advice for two key features of your application: the personal statement and the references.

Part V: Attending Selection Days . . . And Beyond

If a university likes the look of your application, you'll receive an invite to a selection day, where you attend an interview and may sit a test. For many candidates, this is a stressful time. So in this part you'll find plenty of information on what to expect on the day, and how you can make the most of these events and show yourself to be an excellent candidate. I also offer useful advice for the aftermath of the selection day, on how to manage your offers and deal with any disappointments.

Part VI: The Part of Tens

Each chapter in the Part of Tens offers a succinct list of hints, tips and helpful guidance. Head here for quick-grab info on how to make your application stand out and how to avoid common pitfalls throughout the process.

Head to www.dummies.com/extras/getintonursingschooluk for a free bonus Part of Tens chapter. In the bonus chapter, I offer advice on how to stay on top of the associated stress that comes with making a nursing application, to ensure you're in a good position to accept any offers made.

Icons Used in This Book

I use icons throughout the book to draw your attention to information that deserves special attention.

This icon highlights useful ideas or information that can add extra gloss to your preparations and application.

I use this icon to draw your attention to something you should keep in mind.

The Warning icon highlights errors and mistakes that can be very costly and possibly ruin your whole application. Take note!

Where to Go from Here

This book is full to the brim with useful information. Have a flick through the pages and get acquainted with the different sections, and you'll soon appreciate what stage of the application process you're at. You can then decide which chapter to read.

I recommend that you give Part I a go first. You may well know some of this information already, but it does no harm revisiting just who nurses are and what they do – after all, that information forms the very foundation of your application to nursing school.

Remember, you can find free bonus material specific to this book at www.dummies.com/extras/getintonursingschooluk.

Good luck!

Part I

Getting Started with a Career in Nursing

getting started with a career in nursing

In this part . . .

✔ Delve into the history of nursing.

✔ Understand the four different types of nursing: adult, child, mental health and learning disabilities.

✔ Find out about the Nursing and Midwifery Council.

✔ Get familiar with the different places nurses work – from the NHS to the armed forces.

Chapter 1

Getting to Know Nursing

· ·

In This Chapter

▶ Finding out what nursing is

▶ Understanding what a nurse does

▶ Looking at career opportunities

▶ Seeing how you can become a nurse

· ·

*W*elcome to nursing! In this chapter I familiarise you with the nursing profession, delve into a little history and explain the wide-ranging roles nurses carry out. I explain exactly how you train to become a nurse. I also introduce you to the Nursing and Midwifery Council, which crops up frequently throughout this book, the National Health Service and the Royal College of Nursing.

Read on too, to discover how you can travel the world with your valuable nursing skills . . .

Defining the Nursing Profession

What is nursing? Although this looks like a straightforward question, very few candidates can actually answer it well.

The admission tutors expect you to have formed some opinion of what nursing is and how it differs from other healthcare practices. Defining nursing can be difficult because one of its strengths is that it draws together knowledge from many other disciplines, such as the social and biological sciences. The essence of nursing practice is how it utilises a wide range of sources and a mixture of knowledge to create an entirely individual and distinct profession.

Here's an illustration of what nursing is, based upon the Royal College of Nursing's definition:

Nursing is [. . .] the use of clinical judgement in the provision of care to enable people to improve, maintain, or recover health, to cope with health problems, and to achieve the best possible quality of life, whatever their disease or disability, until death.

These are the characteristics that support this definition:

- ✔ **Purpose.** Nurses promote health and wellbeing, minimise suffering and encourage patient understanding. When death is inevitable, nurses offer best-quality care during the end of life.

- ✔ **Intervention.** Nurses encourage patient empowerment and independence by using a unique process to identify nursing needs and offer direct nursing care.

- ✔ **Domain.** Nurses understand how people respond to health and illness, both in the physical and psychological sense but also in social, cultural and spiritual terms too.

- ✔ **Focus.** Nurses focus on patients as a whole and care for all human responses rather than caring for particular conditions or illnesses.

- ✔ **Values.** Nursing is based upon a set of ethical values that respect dignity, autonomy, individuality and the nurse–patient relationship. Nurses accept professional accountability.

- ✔ **Partnership.** Nurses commit to working in partnership with patients, relatives, carers and the multidisciplinary team.

A brief history of nursing

Nursing has been with us through the ages. It may not have been called nursing centuries ago, and it has been associated with wise old women, tribal leaders and even witchcraft at some points in history. However, there have always been individuals ready to come to the aid of others when they are unwell or in distress, and it was often, but not exclusively, women who took on this role of caring.

Nursing is seen as a social construct, responding to current events of the time. Sometimes nursing was the domain of the religious, while in other times it was delegated to the more lowly characters in society. Slowly, nursing became more organised, and although there was little formal education, it was influenced by religious, military and hierarchical structures – which is why nurses have titles such as 'matron', 'sister' and 'staff'.

Prior to the 19th century the portrayal of nursing was one of lower-class women who undertook rather remedial roles in the support of the medical profession, often with little or no training. But modern nursing is, of course, very different (although some modern nurses do use maggots, but that's a story for another time!). So why and how did nursing change?

Today's nursing has its roots in the 19th century and the turbulent times of the Crimean War. Britain was at war with Russia, and as in all wars there was much injury, illness and death. The military had its own medical team made up of doctors and nurses; however, there was much disquiet about the high levels of death among the soldiers. Enter Florence Nightingale – 'the lady with the lamp'.

A truly remarkable person for her times, Florence Nightingale (1820–1910) came from a wealthy family and was very highly educated. She rebelled against conforming to expectations of the well-bred, and instead studied medicine and became renowned for her knowledge of nursing.

She arrived at the British military hospital in Scutari and took over the management of the nurses. She reorganised the care of the wounded and implemented infection control measures such as hand washing with such incredible success that death due to infection was virtually eradicated.

Florence returned to Britain as a national heroine and dedicated the rest of her life to the promotion of nursing. She is recognised as the pioneer of modern nursing and she made a career in nursing respectable for the upper classes. Florence is seen as one of the first nurse researchers and, most importantly for you, championed the formal training of nurses. In 1860 she set up her own nurse training programme at St Thomas's Hospital in London, and much of the training, education and professionalism accepted as normal today is attributed to her vision of nursing.

Florence Nightingale is the most well-known nursing figure, but she is not the only one who has made an impact on nursing. Mary Seacole is well worth researching, as she too nursed during the Crimean War and has been recognised as a nursing pioneer. She was even voted the 'Greatest Black Briton' in 2003.

Nursing is a *profession*, an occupation that requires prolonged training and a formal qualification in a specific subject or science. Professions:

- ✔ Develop specific theoretical knowledge relevant to each different field.

- ✔ Have their own culture.

- ✔ Introduce codes of ethical practice and have legal reinforcement of standards.

- ✔ Offer a service to society and receive public recognition.

- ✔ Receive formal training and have a system of qualification.

- ✔ Require personal autonomy and accountability for practice.

So a professional nurse:

✔ Has undertaken formal education and has achieved a recognised qualification.

✔ Upholds the professional, ethical and legal requirements expected of the profession, and is regulated to do so.

✔ Acts in the best interests of patients and accepts personal accountability for his or her own conduct and behaviour.

Understanding the Role of the Nursing and Midwifery Council

The Nursing and Midwifery Council (NMC) was first set up in 1919 by Parliament (then named the General Nursing Council). The Council:

✔ Works to protect the public and consider their health and wellbeing in all it does.

✔ Sets the standards for education, training and conduct to ensure that nurses deliver high-quality care.

✔ Ensures that nurses continually update their skills and knowledge in order to uphold the professional standards.

✔ Investigates when nurses fall short of meeting the professional standards.

All qualified nurses must register with the NMC in order to practise, and the NMC also plays a role in the selection and education of student nurses. The NMC set the standards for pre-registration education that all universities must comply to. These standards are very lengthy and outline:

✔ Assessment methods to be used to test students.

✔ Different clinical specialities that students must experience.

✔ Guidance on professional expectations of how students should behave.

✔ Principles for the selection of student nurses.

✔ Rules for the length and time that students must be taught.

✔ Skills students much develop (these are grouped into *Essential Skills Clusters*).

You're not expected to fully understand the role of the NMC, but it's highly likely that the admission tutors will refer to them at some point during the selection process, so make sure you have a decent understanding of the organisation's role.

The NMC has specific guidance on how student nurses should conduct themselves. Having some understanding of the professional expectations of students is a good way to impress the admission tutors. Here are some examples of how the NMC expects you to behave as a student nurse, which may be useful in preparing yourself to apply:

✔ Communicate well.

✔ Treat people as individuals and respect their dignity.

✔ Respect a person's right to confidentiality.

✔ Treat all colleagues, team members and all those you work with fairly and without discrimination.

✔ Take responsibility for your own learning.

The NMC website (www.nmc-uk.org) has a section just for student nurses. Use this as a resource.

The Royal College of Nursing

It is worth knowing a little about the Royal College of Nursing (RCN) as, like the NMC, it has a significant role in the support of nursing students. Founded in 1916 as a professional organisation for nurses, the RCN is now recognised as the main trade union for nursing.

The aim of trade unions is to look after the rights and wellbeing of workers, and so the aim of the RCN is to look after nurses, including student nurses. Much of this work is in relation to employment practices such as levels of pay; however the RCN also provides a wealth of other support such as guidelines for practice, a major library of nursing books and journals, financial advice, and, most importantly, support on professional development.

There are alternative trade unions that students can join, but the RCN has been recognised by successive governments (and monarchy, hence the 'Royal') as the 'voice of nursing'.

The RCN website at www.rcn.org.uk is well worth a look. It contains a wealth of information about nursing that can be invaluable in convincing the admission tutors that you understand what being a nursing student means.

For more information on the behaviour expected of you as a student nurse, head to Chapter 5.

Outlining the Role of the Nurse

Nursing is a healthcare profession that focuses on the health and wellbeing of patients, clients and families. But other healthcare professionals, like doctors, physiotherapists and paramedics, do all that too, so what makes nursing special?

What makes nursing a distinct profession with its own identity is that it absorbs elements of all the other healthcare professions and uses them in a unique role. When caring, nurses draw upon knowledge and skill from a wide variety of other disciplines to ensure the patient receives the best care. Nurses spend much more time with patients and clients than any other healthcare professional and they use a range of skills to deliver holistic care. For example, nurses need to know anatomy and physiology in the same way as doctors do, understand and manage medicines like a pharmacist, move and mobilise the patient with similar skills to a physiotherapist, and understand how the client lives in the community like a social worker.

Although nurses don't specialise to the same depth of understanding as these other professions, they're expected to have a thorough and broad understanding and appreciation of all the aspects of the patient's condition. Here are other subjects that nurses need knowledge of to perform their roles:

- ✔ **Law and ethics:** Taking into account patients' rights and beliefs.
- ✔ **Pathophysiology:** Understanding the abnormal function of the body.
- ✔ **Epidemiology:** Knowing the patterns and causes of illness and disease in society.
- ✔ **Politics:** Realising patient choices in a national context.
- ✔ **Psychology:** Appreciating the effects of illness on the patient.
- ✔ **Sociology:** Understanding how society impacts on patients' health.

Nurses use their skills to help and encourage patients to live the life that is normal to them within their own limitations, and where necessary, to allow patients to pass away peacefully and with dignity. They also support families and communities, and work to promote good health and prevent illness in the first place.

Four fields exist in nursing – adult, child, mental health and learning disabilities – and I explore the roles of nurses in these fields in depth in Chapter 2. Depending on their specialty, nurses undertake a wide range of tasks. Here are some you're likely to do as a student nurse:

✔ Apply nursing knowledge to the clinical situation.

✔ Assess patients using nursing models and frameworks.

✔ Deliver nursing care:

- Administering medication

- Bandaging

- Basic life support

- Giving injections

- Recording vital signs such as blood pressure and pulse

- Using technology

- Wound dressing

✔ Give hands-on personal care:

- Bathing and washing

- Eating and drinking

- Moving and walking

- Toileting

✔ Implement care plans and evaluate outcomes.

✔ Offer health promotion.

✔ Plan care that's individualised and appropriate for the patient.

✔ Work with other healthcare professionals.

Within each field the scope of the nurses role and the development of skills and practices are ever-increasing and no two roles are the same. Nurses now have the autonomy and responsibility to care for patients to the level that a few years ago only doctors could do. It is possible today for nurses to have roles that include having their own clinics, making diagnoses of illnesses, undertaking minor surgery and procedures, and prescribing medication.

How your nursing skills and roles develop is dependent on your own career aspirations, your motivation to continue your education and the service development of your field. Table 1-1 shows how a career in nursing can develop. It's based on my own career, and you can see how academic and clinical development has led me to many different roles.

Table 1-1	Example Nurse Career Development	
Date	*Role*	*Qualification*
1985	Student	A-levels
1988	Junior Staff Nurse (Adult Field)	Registered General Nurse
1994	Staff Nurse (Orthopaedics)	Certificate in Supervisory Management
1996	Charge Nurse (Medicine)	Diploma in Professional Practice
2000	Specialist Nurse (Practice Development)	Certificate in Education
2003	Nurse Lecturer (Professional Development)	MSc Research

The staff nurse post is most abundant and is an ideal role for many nurses because it gives an opportunity to develop skills while offering flexibility to manage other commitments.

Examining Who Goes into Nursing

Nursing attracts people of all ages, and it's a career in which you can use your nursing skills right up to retirement (and beyond!). The figures in Table 1-2 show the ages of student nurses and demonstrate the wide range of age groups you'll be working alongside.

Table 1-2	Student Nurse Ages
Age	*Percentage of Student Nursing Population*
18–24	35
25–30	19
31–34	11
35–40	17
41–45	11
46+	7

Younger candidates tend to apply to child nursing, whereas in the other three fields of nursing a pretty even split exists between young and mature students.

Age isn't an issue when applying to nursing – I've offered places to candidates from all of these age ranges. The importance is suitability to nursing and the potential to succeed academically.

What about the male–female ratio? The gender balance in nursing has remained fairly constant for many years, with a greater number of women than men in the profession. Only 11 per cent of nurses are men. In both mental health nursing and learning disabilities nursing you find a higher percentage of men than in adult fields, and the child field has the lowest number of men of all fields.

If you're a man reading this book, don't be fooled into believing you can't nurse in all fields. The stereotyping that led men to favour one field over the other is very much redundant now, and you'll be fully accepted – indeed encouraged – to follow your heart and apply for the field that best suits you and your skills.

Seeing Where Nurses Work

Each government of the four UK countries sets its own health agenda, and this shapes how many nurses are needed based on population, illness and changing health provision. The good news is that nurses are in demand and significant numbers are needed to support the healthcare system. Table 1-3 shows the number of nurses registered with the NMC for 2011. You can see that as well as many thousands of nurses working throughout the UK, 26,000 UK nurses work abroad.

Table 1-3	Numbers of Nurses in the UK
Location of Nurses	*Numbers*
England	531,000
Scotland	70,000
Wales	34,000
Northern Ireland	23,000
NMC registered nurses working outside the UK	26,000

Just because England has the greatest number of nurses doesn't mean that this is where you'll find the greatest number of opportunities. All countries have equal needs from nursing based on their population size and health requirements, so don't feel that you must move to new areas to secure the best roles.

When working within the UK, you have a choice of several settings, as I outline in the following sections.

The National Health Service

The NHS is by far the largest organisation with the greatest number and variety of roles for nurses of all fields. It's the largest single employer in the UK with over 1.7 million people looking after a population of nearly 62 million people – the NHS is kept very busy! The main provider of healthcare for the general population, the NHS undoubtedly has a role or speciality to suit your interest. If you need to have a job closer to home, but with good opportunity to develop your skills and expertise, then the NHS has much to offer.

Here are the more usual clinical areas in which NHS nurses work:

- ✔ **Hospitals.** These may be large specialist centres that look after patients with a range of conditions, offering palliative care, medicine and surgery, and catering to elderly, mentally ill and other types of patient. Or they may be small community hospitals with just a few buildings that look after patients for respite or rehabilitative care. Nurses work in day centres, wards and departments such as X-ray or endoscopy. Most of the larger hospitals have the full range of services available, so patients can undertake tests, investigations and operations all on the same site.

- ✔ **In the community.** Nurses provide care within the healthcare system or alongside other public services. Examples include working in GP practices or medical centres, working with children in schools and with offenders within the justice system, and working alongside social care services. Some also nurse patients in their own homes.

To get a feel for what the NHS can do for your career, take a look at their career planner on the NHS careers website: http://nursingcareers.nhsemployers.org.

NHS pay scales

NHS pay scales are arranged nationally for the public sector, and there are yearly negotiations between the government, employers and unions to decide on any future increases or changes to working arrangements. While nursing won't make you rich, the levels of pay are consistent with other public sector roles.

Choosing a particular field of nursing doesn't offer pay advantages; all fields are banded the same against their roles. Selecting the right field and progressing your career does more for increasing your pay than attempting to predict now which field will result in better financial rewards.

If you want to know how much you'll be paid as a nurse, check out the NHS jobs website at www.jobs.nhs.uk. This site is great for indicating the types of jobs on offer and rates of pay.

The independent sector

The independent sector is expanding very rapidly, and it has become an important partner to the NHS. Whereas traditionally it was seen as caring for old age or cosmetic surgery, it now offers services that complement NHS ones. Often patients from the NHS are cared for by nurses in the independent sector, and so many of the skills nurses develop are transferrable between the different employers.

Nurses in the independent sector work in a range of settings:

- **Private hospitals** tend to specialise in surgical procedures, and while cosmetic surgery is an important aspect of their healthcare, private hospitals carry out many other kinds of surgery. These hospitals have state-of-the-art equipment and technology and so can offer a lot of care surrounding health assessments. Many of these hospitals provide care for NHS patients as well as private ones. If, for example, NHS waiting lists are too long for a particular specialty, the care provision is purchased from the local private hospital.

- **Residential and nursing homes** are for people who need care on a 24-hours-a-day basis, but not in a hospital. Residential homes can be for adults, children or people with learning disabilities, and they often have nurses with the relevant experience, but the patients don't always require nursing care. Nursing homes are for those people who require 24-hour nursing care.

✓ **Charities** can employ nurses to help within their organisations; for example, cancer charities offer nursing care to the public, especially in the palliative stages of the illness. Nurses are employed for their specialised knowledge and offer very individualised care, either at care centres or the patient's own home.

✓ **Businesses** employ occupational health nurses who have specific knowledge and skills in workplace practice and health and safety issues. One of their primary roles is to ensure employees are fit and healthy to undertake or return to their jobs.

The armed forces

Opportunities exist to spend some of your nursing career within the armed forces. But the fields of nursing are limited, with many more opportunities for adult nurses than, say, learning disability nurses, and depending on which of the forces you choose, the clinical environment and nursing skills can be quite different – from field hospitals in battle zones abroad to hospitals in the UK.

Check out the websites for each of the three armed forces at:

✓ **RAF:** www.raf.mod.uk/careers/jobs/nursing officer.cfm

✓ **Army:** www.army.mod.uk/army-medical-services/ 9869.aspx

✓ **Navy:** www.qarnns.co.uk

These websites provide information on career progression and opportunities for qualified and student nurses.

Voluntary services

You may want to use your skills to help people in a voluntary capacity. Many organisations need nurses to support their projects in the poorer regions of the world. These organisations usually require physical nursing skills and some experience in tropical medicine, but there are opportunities for many children's and adult nurses.

The following organisations' websites have some very useful information about volunteering as a nurse:

- ✓ **Voluntary Services Overseas (VSO):** www.vso.org.uk/
- ✓ **Medecins Sans Frontieres:** www.msf.org.uk/
- ✓ **Projects Abroad:** www.projects-abroad.co.uk/

Nursing overseas

If you want to spread your wings, consider the many opportunities to use your nursing skills abroad. The figure of 26,000 nurses working outside the UK demonstrates that NMC-registered nurses are appreciated throughout the world.

It's quite possible to spend a good period of your career gaining short-term employment on (usually) two-year contracts with nursing organisations in other countries. The ability to move from country to country, using your skills and seeing new cultures while being paid handsomely is very attractive to some nurses.

If you want to nurse abroad, consider that once you've completed your nurse education you need a few years' experience before many countries will offer you jobs. Some countries also require you to sit a state exam.

Many websites advertise jobs abroad. However, each country has its own rules and regulations, so use a licensed agency when making plans for overseas employment.

Training to Become a Nurse

So how do you become a nurse? Well, you do a three-year degree in nursing at a university, in which you spend half your time on academic learning and the rest in clinical practice.

Each subsequent chapter in this book leads you through the process, but to start you off, here's an overview.

1. Achieve the necessary academic qualifications.

Nursing students need a good foundation from compulsory education and higher academic qualifications for universities to seriously consider their application. Chapter 3 reviews the qualifications that support your application.

2. Be fit to practise.

Nursing demands only the best from its nursing students, and in your application you must meet professional requirements in areas like health and criminal record. Chapter 4 takes you through each of the different professional aspects and helps you understand how fitness to practise applies to you.

3. Ensure you demonstrate the necessary personal attributes.

Personal development is as important as academic qualifications, and in Chapter 5 I explain the different characteristics of a good nursing student. Having the right attitude and displaying the correct behaviours makes a significant difference to the quality of care that patients receive.

4. Gain care experience.

Universities are interested in how you demonstrate that care and compassion are focal to the way you behave and also want to know that you have good communication and teamwork skills. Nurses do not work alone, and they require good interpersonal skills to ensure that patients receive the right care, not only from the nurses themselves but from the rest of the healthcare team. Developing these skills takes time, and you need to consider whether gaining care experience is useful to help demonstrate your abilities. Chapter 6 tells you all you need to know about care experience.

5. Research universities and courses.

You may already have in mind a university you want to go to, perhaps the one local to home or another with a good reputation. On the other hand you may not yet have thought about universities and their role in you becoming a nurse. Researching universities and finding the right course for you takes some effort. Chapters 7 and 8 go into detail on how to weigh up different unis and their courses, and Chapter 9 helps you make the best of visits to unis.

You can choose up to five different courses or universities. In fact, I encourage you to consider more than one option. As I talk you through the different aspects of selecting your choices you see that finding out about each university isn't as simple as reading a prospectus. Be prepared for a bit of travelling and a little detective work!

6. Check you have finance in place.

In Chapter 10 I take you through money matters. Too often candidates begin the application process and then discover, down the road, that they can't afford to study. Check out Chapter 10 to ensure you've thought of all the financial aspects.

7. **Submit your application form.**

   You apply for a university place through the Universities and Colleges Admissions Service (UCAS), and I explain the UCAS process in Chapter 11. The application comprises your personal statement (Chapter 12) and references (Chapter 13).

Submitting the best application possible is essential in getting yourself noticed by the admissions tutors. They are the people who make decisions about your application and who offer you a place or decide that on this occasion you have been successful. The goal at this point is to present yourself (on paper) in such a way that the admissions tutors want to see you and invite you to interview.

8. **Attend selection days.**

   Many universities use a series of interviews and/or tests to assess your suitability for nursing, and you need to spend some time preparing for these. Chapter 14 helps you understand the selection process, and Chapters 15 and 16 prepare you for assessments and interviews, respectively. Testing is used to make sure that you have the correct abilities and behaviours to begin a nursing programme; having the right attitude regarding people, being able to calculate numbers and having good communication skills are all essential.

   The NMC like all nursing students to have been seen by the admissions team before an offer is made. The fact that you have been invited to meet the team is good news as it now allows you to show off your abilities in person. This stage of the application process is undoubtedly the most stressful, and chapter 14 helps explain what happens on these days.

9. **Deal with the results.**

   Getting onto a nursing course is a competitive process. I hope that after reading this book and making solid preparations you have some positive offers from your choices of university. Chapter 17 explains how offers are made, what the terminology means and how to proceed when you receive offers or rejections.

If you're a little confused by all the whens and what fors of putting your application together, Table 1-4 gives a summary:

Table 1-4	Summary of Nursing Training
Year 1	
May	Think about your A-level or course choices. University might be 2 years away but you have to take advice to enroll now on the right subjects.
September	Start your two-year course. Think also about gaining some nursing experience.
Year 2	
April	If you're considering a one-year course such as ACCESS start making enquiries about enrolment for September.
June	Do your research on universities and their open days.
July	Open day events normally start now and you want to make your visits before applying.
September	Continue with the second year of your course or start your one-year course.
October	Begin to work on your application form.
November	Have your application form ready so your referee can complete their section.
Year 3	
January	If you haven't sent your application to UCAS yet, be quick or you'll miss the deadline date (usually 15 January).
February	Decisions start to be made by the admissions team and invites to selection events start arriving.
March	You should have attended any interviews by now.
April	Universities have made most of their decisions and you have some offers.
May	Time to make your decisions – which offer to accept (usually 8 May).
August	Course results are announced. If you made the grade the universities confirm your place on their programme.
October	You start your nursing programme.

Getting to university is a long, hard process that may be a few years in the planning. But knowing that when you step onto campus you're starting the journey into a profession that leads to meeting wonderful people and making lifelong friends is a wonderful feeling.

Chapter 2

Exploring Your Options: Nursing Fields

*N*urses specialise in four fields: adult, child, mental health and learning disabilities. Before logging on to your computer and filling out your application form for nursing, you need to make sure that you fully understand your chosen field and are sure it's the right path for you. After you start your nurse training, you'll find changing course difficult, so you're best making the right decision now. And in this chapter I help you do just that, by outlining the different types of nurses and their roles and responsibilities.

 Some universities won't allow you to apply to more than one field of nursing. Check with your chosen university before sending off your application form. And be aware that although other universities allow multiple field applications, because you submit only one personal statement across your choices, the lack of specialism in your application may hinder your chances of success.

Looking at the Nursing Field Ratios

Each of the nursing fields recruits nurses in relation to the amount of patients, the type of conditions and the way in which care is delivered. Adult nursing is the most in demand and has the most places, whereas learning disabilities is a very specialist role and recruits fewer nurses. Table 2-1 shows UK figures for nurse employment in 2011.

Nursing: Vocation, not job

In its basic definition a *job* is work that is undertaken for which you receive pay; the job could be, for example, cleaning windows or gardening or working as a shop assistant. You could consider nursing to be a job – you carry out tasks for which you receive. But nursing is much more. Very few nurses stay in the same role, have limited responsibilities and leave the job at 'the bedside' when they clock off, and most nurses don't enter nursing because of the pay. Nursing becomes part of who you are, and it very much impacts other parts of your life. For many, nursing is a vocation that becomes a lifelong career.

Table 2-1	UK Figures for Nurse Recruitment, 2011
Field	*Number of Nurses Employed*
Adult	608,000
Mental health	100,000
Child	41,000
Learning disabilities	24,000

Don't let the difference in numbers influence your choice of nursing fields. Each field has a wide range of roles and specialties that allow a fulfilling career. You may well come to regret your decision if you choose a field of nursing based on how many nurses there are.

Adult Nursing

Adult nursing is by far the largest field of nursing. This is hardly surprising when you consider the nature of the role. Adult nurses care for patients from late teenage years right through until old age, and not only is this a large age group but the type of nursing is also very expansive.

Recognising the scope of adult nursing

Think about just how many areas adult nurses cover:

✔ **Specific parts of the body:** Consider the human body. Looking at the head alone, think of the different basic features – skull, brain, eyes, ears, nose, teeth, skin and hair. Each of these body parts can go wrong – be injured or become unwell – and then the patient needs nursing. In the case of the head, several nurses can help: the neurological nurse (brain), ophthalmic nurse (eyes), ENT nurse (ear, nose and throat), dental nurse (teeth) and dermatology nurse (skin), just to name a few. Apply the same thinking to the rest of the body, with all its organs, muscles and bones, and you start to get an understanding of how many different types of nurses there can be focusing on specific parts.

✔ **Specific conditions and treatments:** Complications may require treatment through surgery or a medical approach, and in some cases, when treatments aren't going to improve the condition, a patient needs a palliative approach to care. Therefore, there are nurses for different conditions or treatments, such as the heamatology nurse, the theatre nurse, the diabetic nurse and the oncology nurse.

✔ **Critical and long-term care:** Complications to the body can arise in very different ways. Patients can suffer from acute symptoms due to trauma, such as a traffic accident, or sudden-onset illness, such as a heart attack. Other illnesses are long lasting, or *chronic*, where the patient has to live with the condition and adapt her lifestyle to accommodate it; examples of such illnesses include stroke, arthritis and asthma. So some nurses work in critical care, and others work in long-term care.

Understanding the role of the adult nurse

The focus of adult nursing is on the patient rather than the illness or disease. This means the nurse approaches the care from the patient's perspective and not from a medical perspective. The intention is to ensure that the patient understands the illness and see how the illness impacts on the patient's everyday activities. The nurse then plans and delivers nursing care with the patient's problems as a core to the interventions.

The care a nurse provides is *holistic care*, because the nurse addresses the patient as a whole and doesn't focus only on the illness or disease.

One of the main roles of the nurse is to support patients to carry out daily activities like washing, going to the toilet, eating and drinking, working, playing and socialising. These activities affect how the patient relates to her illness, and when the activities are neglected, the patient struggles to cope. This is *fundamental care*, also known as basic nursing care, and it underpins every other aspect of the adult nurse's practice.

Adult nurses work as part of a multidisciplinary team and act as the patient's advocate to ensure that all healthcare professionals are clear about the patient's expectations, concerns and wishes. It's usual for nurses to be the voice of the patient when working with medical staff, physiotherapists, occupational therapists, social workers and many other members of the healthcare team.

Although fundamental care is the foundation for good nursing care, adult nurses also need an extensive understanding of health and social care. The complexity of the adult nurse's roles requires her to have a range of skills appropriate to her clinical specialism, and it isn't unusual for nurses to undertake roles that are traditionally the domain of doctors, such as making clinical diagnosis, treating wounds and prescribing medication.

Seeing where adult nurses work

Adult nurses work in a range of clinical settings in both the public and private sectors:

- ✔ **Hospitals.** Most hospitals are large, specialised buildings that offer a wide range of services and it is typical for nurses to work in wards, departments and care units:

  - **Wards.** Nurses work in medical wards where the focus is on particular illnesses such as diabetes, cardiac or respiratory conditions. Other types of wards can include respite care where patients are nursed for short periods of time to help families or rehabilitation wards where nurses work with the patients to promote independence before going home. Nurses also work in surgical wards: those that cover a range of surgical procedures and specialist wards that focus on specific types of surgery such as neurosurgery, orthopaedics or gynaecology.

  - **Specialist units.** These areas, such as intensive care, accident and emergency or theatre nursing, deliver very specialised care, often when patients have unstable or acute conditions and need very close monitoring.

  - **Departments and units.** Many hospitals have departments that offer nursing care but not in typical ward environments – for example, day centres, where patients with strokes or dementia receive rehabilitation care. Other examples include the outpatients department or day surgery units where patients have investigations and minor procedures.

✔ **The community.** Adult nurses work in the community in a variety of settings, including district nursing, liaison nursing or in GP practices. They visit patients in their own homes or work out of health centres.

✔ **Industry.** Many nurses have a career working in organisations that don't have a healthcare emphasis. For example, many nurses work in occupational health and are employed by large companies to look after the health and wellbeing of the other employees. Another example is the role of in-flight nursing, where the nurse uses their skills on board airlines to repatriate the sick back to their home.

Looking at key tasks

Adult nurses have a wide range of skills developed according to their specialist areas. All adult nurses have skills in fundamental nursing and are expected to:

✔ Act as advocate for the patient in team meetings.

✔ Check and administer drugs including injections.

✔ Communicate with patients, families and carers.

✔ Educate and promote health.

✔ Mentor students.

✔ Perform nursing assessments and identify patients' needs.

✔ Perform observations and record blood pressure, pulse, respirations and temperature.

✔ Perform wound dressing and remove sutures.

✔ Write care plans and maintain legal documentation.

Children's Nursing

In child nursing the age group is very diverse, from newborn babies to older teenagers. This age group represents approximately 20 per cent of the population but counts disproportionately for those who use the healthcare service, especially in relation to injury and emergency care.

Children aren't 'little adults'; they have their own health needs distinct from those of adults that require specialist nurses. The children's nurse works not only with the child but also closely with the parents or carers.

Children suffer from a catalogue of acute and long-term illnesses and medical conditions in much the same way as adults do, but the impact of how the disease affects children can be very different. Children are vulnerable individuals and need to be treated with sensitivity and understanding. The young have difficulty communicating their worries and anxieties, and it takes special training and consideration to ensure that nursing care is appropriate.

Understanding the role of the children's nurse

The emphasis in children's nursing is family-centred care and the recognition that children are best cared for by their parents or those they know well.

A children's nurse must:

- ✔ **Act as the child's advocate.** The nurse puts the best interest of the child first, protecting her from abuse and neglect, and ensuring her views and preferences are taken into account.

- ✔ **Understand the biological, psychological and social aspects that affect children.** In particular, the nurse understands stages of human development and how to care for children as they grow up, in terms of the cultural, physical and mental concerns of the child.

- ✔ **Communicate and assess expertly.** Children's nurses face a range of complex and unpredictable situations where sound clinical judgments are necessary to manage rapidly deteriorating situations or ethically challenging occurrences, especially when caring for infants and young children.

- ✔ **Handle technology.** The nurse embraces new innovations and is competent in the use of technology. Safe and effective care of children and young people, especially those ill and disabled, relies considerably on the nurse's ability to complement her nursing skills with medical aids and equipment.

- ✔ **Work well with others.** You're expected to be involved with the multidisciplinary team and place the child's interest first when working with medical practitioners, physiotherapists, occupational therapists, psychologists and social workers. This requires good leadership skills, a professional attitude and the ability to challenge views and opinions.

Seeing where children's nurses work

Your working environment depends upon your role. Health provision is gradually moving to a more community-based service, but some care can't be delivered near to or in the child's own home, and hospital-based care is still a significant part of children's nursing.

Here's where children's nurses work:

- ✔ **Hospital.** You find children's nurses in various locations of a hospital, such as:

  - **Neonatal intensive care.** Neonatal nurses care for newborn babies who are born prematurely or who are unwell. Many causes of illness in the newborn are compounded by the immature development of the baby and require specialist intensive care. Neonatal nurses are highly trained and have a very close working relationship with the multidisciplinary team.

  - **Children's ward.** Many hospitals have children's wards that care for a variety of conditions both medical and surgical. Nurses on children's wards care for children who require surgical intervention, either from physical conditions such as appendicitis or due to traumatic injury due to an accident. They also care for children with medical conditions including asthma, cystic fibrosis and respiratory infections. These wards often also have separate units for caring on a short-stay basis, such as oncology or diabetes units.

  - **Adult areas.** Some hospitals have specialist children's nurses working in departments and units that may not be immediately recognised as children's: for example, dermatology units and accident and emergency departments or in theatre recovery. These are highly experienced children's nurses with additional training in their chosen specialty.

- ✔ **Community.** Children's nurses in the community aim to offer care in the child's own home. Many children with life-limiting or terminal conditions, complex disabilities and long-term conditions such as asthma and eczema are able to live and be cared for at home. Community nursing requires skill and experience at managing complex conditions and working independently within a multidisciplinary team.

- ✔ **School.** It's possible to gain a role as a school nurse straight after your initial registration, but normally these nurses undertake a specialist practice qualification. School nurses are responsible for providing health and sex education, managing illnesses at school, undertaking developmental screening and administering immunisation programmes.

Looking at key tasks

Although duties will vary according to the role, all children's nurses have fundamental skills in practical procedures, such as:

✔ Administering drugs and giving injections.

✔ Assessing patients and planning effective care.

✔ Cleaning and dressing wounds.

✔ Enabling children to socialise and play.

✔ Giving psychological care to reduce stress and anxiety.

✔ Helping children eat and drink.

✔ Helping children with their personal hygiene.

✔ Measuring temperatures and taking blood pressures.

✔ Using health promotion strategies to encourage good health and wellbeing.

✔ Working closely with family and carers and demonstrating excellent communication skills.

Mental Health Nursing

Mental health is of serious concern. Aside from the misery of mental illness itself, statistics demonstrate that those with a mental health problem encounter more negative life experiences, such as unemployment, physical illness and social discrimination, than that of the general population. The issue is increasingly common, with an estimated one in four people experiencing a mental health condition at some point in their lives.

There's a growing recognition that the mental health of individuals has been long neglected, and the government is currently developing policies to improve medical care in this area. To implement such policies the country needs a competent and professional mental health nursing staff with the necessary knowledge and skills.

Defining mental health

The World Health Organisation suggests that to be healthy does not necessarily require the absence of disease or illness but to be in a state of complete physical, mental and social wellbeing. *Mental health*, therefore, broadly relates to the cognitive and emotional capabilities of the person to be able to meet the everyday demands of living.

Many problems are covered by the term 'mental illness'; here are some that a mental health nurse commonly deals with:

- ✔ **Attention deficit hyperactive disorder (ADHD)** is character-ised by difficulties with inattention, hyperactivity and impul-siveness. It's the most prevalent childhood disorder, and symptoms include the child being easily distracted, struggling to concentrate on what she's doing or saying and becoming very restless and fidgety.

- ✔ **Bipolar,** also known as manic depression, causes severe mood swings in patients. Although emotions are never con-stantly stable in patients with bipolar, the change in moods are exaggerated from low, depressive periods to highly over-active emotions. These changes in moods can last several weeks to several months.

- ✔ **Dementia** is a syndrome in which the patient gradually loses brain function, particularly in the areas of memory, think-ing, language, understanding and judgment. Many types of dementia exist, but the most well-known type is Alzheimer's. Dementia is a common condition, and the number of cases is likely to double over the next 30 years as people live longer.

- ✔ **Obsessive compulsive disorder (OCD)** is associated with obsessive thoughts and compulsive behaviour. The obsession can be both frightening and unpleasant and usually takes over many aspects of the patient's life. The condition is relatively common, with an estimated 3–5 people in every 100 being affected.

- ✔ **Schizophrenia** is a psychotic illness that causes hallucina-tions and/or delusions that can cause a change in behav-iour. Often the patient can't differentiate between her own thoughts and ideas and reality. The common perception that all schizophrenics have split personalities and are violent is untrue; schizophrenics are more likely to be victims than perpetrators of violence.

- ✔ **Substance misuse** can affect a patient's mental health, espe-cially if they already suffer from a mental health condition. Society is tolerant of substance use, and smoking, alcohol and recreational drugs are still largely accepted lifestyle choices. Substance *misuse*, however, is when the drugs have a negative effect on a person's functioning.

Understanding the role of the mental health nurse

In very broad terms, mental health nurses look after the psychological care of the patient.

As a mental health nurse you work with patients who suffer from mental health issues with the intention to help them recover from their illness or come to terms with how to live with their illness. Caring for the patient also includes supporting and encouraging the family to participate in the care. Mental health nurses are involved with identifying the psychological condition and any associated physical issues, the assessments of the patient's problems, and the management of any drug regime used to control the condition.

Mental health nurses care for patients from all backgrounds, cultures and ages, including children.

Mental health nurses rely on their skill at communication and strength of personality as core attributes when helping patients. Often a patient's condition can mean their behaviour is very manipulative or demanding and the role of the nurse is to see these as symptoms and manage these episodes by using a range of communication skills that allow a partnership to develop between the patient and the nurse.

Another role of the mental health nurse is to offer empathy to the patient and be non-judgemental with regard to the patient's behaviour or condition. The nurse acts as the patient's advocate, breaking down misconceptions within the general public and helping to improve the image of mental health in society.

Seeing where mental health nurses work

Mental health nurse are involved with patients' care in the following settings:

> ✔ **The community.** The community mental health team provides assessment and care co-ordination for those people who have severe or enduring mental health problems. Based in the community, the nurses visit patients in their own homes and residential settings. (Residential homes contain patients who've been assessed as needing full 24-hour care and would

be at risk living in their own homes, but don't require hospital admission.) The team is multidisciplinary, and nurses work alongside psychiatrists, social workers, psychologists and occupational therapists.

✔ **Institutional settings.** These are environments for people with a very high level of offending and challenging behaviour. The patients present a danger to others and themselves and are often in the criminal justice system. You work in a secure setting such as a prison, police station or court.

✔ **Mental health hospitals.** Once all mental health patients lived locked away in institutions – think dreary stone buildings on hillsides away from the population. But many of the hospitals now are new purpose-built developments. They cater for people who have been detained under the Mental Health Act and require a secure setting. Nurses in these settings deal with acute disorders, delivering effective care and assessing care pathways to promote health and wellbeing. Typical types of ward include acute admissions wards, where patients need initial assessments of their problems, or long-term wards where patients who have become institutionalised and cannot manage living in the community are nursed.

Looking at key tasks

The daily activities of the mental health nurse relate to the psychological care of the person; a significant difference to the 'hands-on' care delivered by adult and children's nurses. But depending on the type of patient, mental health nurses may also help on the physical side too, such as when nursing elderly mentally ill patients who have considerable physical health needs.

Here are some of the typical roles of the nurse:

✔ Acting as the patient's advocate and ensuring legal requirements are met.

✔ Administering medication, including injections, and monitoring effects.

✔ Applying calming techniques in the management of emotions and behaviours, including watching clients who are at risk of self-harming.

✔ Assessing the patient's mental health and talking to the patient about her problems.

✔ Building relationships, fostering trust and interpreting needs.

✔ Organising care plans to develop the patient's social skills.

✔ Physical care dependent upon the patient, such as personal hygiene, eating, drinking and mobility.

✔ Using high-level communication skills to respond to distressed patients.

✔ Working with families and carers to promote understanding of mental health issues and encourage acceptance.

Learning Disabilities Nursing

The least well known of the four nursing fields, learning disabilities nursing, aims to support the wellbeing and social inclusion of people with learning disabilities. Learning disabilities affect up to 2 per cent of the UK population, and they're lifelong conditions. Advances in healthcare and greater understanding of the conditions has brought about an improvement in the health and wellbeing of people with learning disabilities, but the number of children and adults diagnosed is increasing, and with it the need for appropriately trained nurses.

Defining learning disabilities

Learning disabilities affect a person's ability to learn, to communicate and to carry out everyday tasks. More specifically, people with learning disabilities have core difficulties in understanding what is being said to them but also expressing their own needs. They often find it difficult to cope with change and see life events in a very different way to others, and they can have memory and attention issues as well.

To compound these difficulties, many people with learning disabilities also have significant physical disabilities that can often lead to premature death. Due to their difficulties with communication and everyday tasks, social isolation can often occur, with the patient having little involvement with mainstream society.

It's not always apparent that someone has a learning disability, but two features are outwardly suggestive:

✔ **Autism** is referred to as a *spectrum condition* because it varies quite considerably in how it affects each person. Autism causes problems with communication and many patients have difficulty with the usual modes of verbal and non-verbal communication. There are also issues with social interaction, with patients lacking the social skills needed to engage and maintain relationships; some may actively seek social interaction while others withdraw from social activity. People with autism are also very rigid in how they perceive concepts and lack imagination; this causes issues with abstract situations such as understanding emotions.

✔ **Challenging behaviour** is a term used to explain behaviour that, due to its intensity and duration, causes concern for the safety of the patient or others. Causes for the behaviour are quite numerous but may stem from mental health, abuse, poor housing or physical discomfort. In a small number of people the behaviour leads to criminal offences, and these patients often need support from the learning disability services while they are being reviewed by the justice system.

Understanding the role of the learning disabilities nurse

People with learning disabilities have very complex problems and are more susceptible to poorer physical, social and psychological wellbeing than that of the ordinary population. Learning disabilities nurses act as advocates for patients and help them as follows:

✔ **Physical.** Nurses address the personal care of the patient, such as washing and dressing, and may also help with eating and drinking if the patient has swallowing problems. Many patients suffer sensory impairments, such as deafness and visual problems, and those with Down's syndrome are more susceptible to infections such as pneumonia. Epilepsy affects approximately a third of people with a learning disability and is often associated with hospitalisation due to the severity or social isolation from anxiety. The role of the nurse here is to support both personal care but also manage a range of clinical conditions such as chest infections or epilepsy.

✔ **Psychological.** Nurses implement strategies that enhance self-care, peer support and risk of self-harm. People with learning disabilities have poor coping mechanisms, find it difficult to manage situations and suffer from poor self-esteem, often because of discrimination. These patients can become very dependent upon others and particularly their helpers and nurses.

✔ **Social.** People with learning disabilities can become isolated from society because they lack the skills to form relationships, which can lead to them mixing with inappropriate peer groups. Many people with learning disabilities live with their families, but others live in residential settings, which may exacerbate their problems by encouraging them to become institutionalised. Learning disabilities nurses develop strategies with patients, families, social services and other agencies to enable social inclusion.

Seeing where learning disabilities nurses work

Historically, people with learning disabilities were segregated from society in large institutions, but most people now live in community settings, either independently or with support, and only the most severe cases are in-patients.

- ✔ **The community.** Many nurses work as part of community teams with the intention of keeping people with learning disabilities within their local community and encouraging inclusion wherever possible. Mild symptoms affect over three quarters of patients, and the majority have independent lives, have families, gain employment and require the services of the learning disabilities nurse only in times of crisis. Moderate symptoms require a higher level of support and these patients have difficulty communicating their needs and handling every-day tasks. They often live with their parents, have every-day support and require help from a number of health and social services, but some live in residential accommodation or attend day services where independence is encouraged.

  The community teams are made up of many healthcare professionals, and learning disabilities nurses work alongside occupational therapists, physiotherapists, psychiatrists, social workers and speech and language therapists.

- ✔ **Specialist care units.** In more severe cases of learning disabilities the person may require nursing in a specialist in-patient accommodation, which may be part of a large hospital or a purpose-built unit. The more severe and profound the symptoms, such as self-injury and challenging behaviour, the greater the patient's needs. These units care for patients who have a more complex level of disability or need acute management for epilepsy.

Due to the expansive spectrum of learning disabilities, nurses are required to work in close partnership with other nurses and agencies, most notably mental health nursing and social work. Collaborative working is an essential function for the learning disabilities nurse, who may find herself working as part of the social services team or within a mental health environment such as a forensic secure unit.

Looking at key tasks

Learning disabilities nurses focus on ensuring the patient is able to integrate into society and to lead a normal life. This social model of care means that the nurse spends a considerable amount of time promoting health, developing relationships and enabling access to support mechanisms, as well as ensuring physical wellbeing.

The job description includes:

✔ Carrying out group work aimed at encouraging behaviour management and healthy living.

✔ Encouraging equality and equal access to community and public services.

✔ Interpreting and understanding behaviours in patients.

✔ Liaising with hospital staff for planned admissions for health-care needs.

✔ Managing and coordinating health needs such as epilepsy, dental problems, swallowing problems and respiratory infections.

✔ Planning activities and social events in supported living settings.

✔ Using expert communication skills to engage with vulnerable patients.

✔ Working in a multidisciplinary team to advocate for individuals

Separating Nursing Fields from Other Professions

With all healthcare professions, inevitably some roles overlap. The overlap helps each profession understand the roles and respon-sibilities of others, which promotes good working relationships. However, each profession has its distinct culture and values, which stand apart from those of others.

Make sure you don't muddle up roles from nursing with roles from other professions. The following sections help you avoid common areas of confusion.

Midwifery versus children's nursing

A *midwife* is a qualified professional who cares for the emotional, physical and psychological processes of pregnancy and birth. Midwives are regulated by the Nursing and Midwifery Council (NMC) and they undertake a professional education programme that's similar to the nursing programme. But they are *not* nurses and they apply a different philosophy of care to their clients.

Many candidates are undecided between being a midwife or a children's nurse and associate the two as being similar. There is some relationship between the professions when referring to neonatal care or the very young baby; however, the role of the midwife in care of the baby stops after the postnatal period. Should a young baby require care she's more likely to be nursed by a children's nurse than a midwife. Candidates often like the idea of looking after small babies but are unsure what this means.

In a nutshell: midwives predominately look after women and children's nurses look after children of all ages.

Social work versus learning disabilities nursing

Social work centres around people and their communities and deals with social problems like poverty and discrimination. The intention of social workers is to improve the quality of life and wellbeing of individuals, groups or communities that are afflicted with real or perceived social injustices.

Social workers work with a variety of clients, such as:

- ✔ Adults with learning disabilities
- ✔ People who are socially excluded
- ✔ People with substance addictions
- ✔ Refugees and asylum seekers
- ✔ Vulnerable children
- ✔ Vulnerable older people
- ✔ Young offenders

Notice the first item on that list – adults with learning disabilities. A significant part of the learning disabilities nurse's role is to ensure acceptance and integration of the patient into society. The close working relationship with social services means that the social role of the two professions is similar if not identical. But the nurse role has professional responsibilities in relation to the NMC and a physical caring aspect is present in the nurse's role that is not part of social work.

You need to have a clear understanding of whether it's the nursing or the social aspect that's brought learning disabilities to your attention. If you're undecided, some universities offer a dual registration qualification: after 4 years of university education you're eligibile to register as both a learning disability nurse and a social worker.

Care work versus nursing

Care work encompasses caring for a loved one and working as a nursing auxiliary or support worker who helps registered health-care professionals perform their daily activities. A care worker *isn't* a registered nurse; care workers give informal care, though they may have undertaken vocational training.

Many candidates apply to nursing after undertaking care experiences but have little appreciation of the differences between the carer and professional. When asked at interview to describe the differences between a carer and a qualified nurse, their answer relates to tasks like undertaking drugs rounds and liaising with the doctors to completing the documentation. Very few candidates see the wider implications and recognise the responsibilities and behaviours necessary in nursing for clinical decision-making, management of risk and assessment of the patients, and the level of underpinning knowledge that goes with professional registration.

 I often ask at interview what the difference is between a care worker feeding a patient and a nurse feeding a patient. I expect the care worker to feed competently and ensure the patient has had enough to eat. The nurse, however, needs to assess the patient's ability to eat and digest the food, understand the nutritional content of the food in relation to the patient's condition and be assessing the patient's skin for sores, any elimination difficulties, and the mental wellbeing of the patient.

 Caring is an element of nursing, but it's not the sum total of nursing. Nursing care is more advanced than personal care and requires better skills, knowledge and professionalism. Although many carers develop the right attitude and become excellent nurses, not all have the commitment or aptitude to develop to the level of a nurse.

Part II

Focusing on Your Personal Development

Top Five Qualities in a Nurse

- ✔ **Care.** Through their whole lives patients expect to receive care that's consistently of high quality. The nurse demonstrates care through clinical skills and also behaviour and attitude.

- ✔ **Compassion.** Developing relationships built on empathy, kindness, respect and dignity leads to compassionate care. Nurses are expected to demonstrate skills of delivering care that promotes trust and understanding with the patient.

- ✔ **Competence.** Nurses must have the knowledge, skills and attitude to provide good-quality care that's supported by the best available evidence. Having the capability to use research and evidence in care delivery is an important aspect of nursing.

- ✔ **Communication.** Having good communication skills is about appreciating the patient's view of his health problems and responding in a manner that reflects the patient's concerns and allows the patient to make decisions. Nurses should also demonstrate good inter-professional communication skills as well.

- ✔ **Courage.** In the context of nursing, courage relates to the ability to manage difficult situations and speak up when things are wrong, to ensure that patients receive the right care. This may involve reporting another practitioner to their mentor or a member of the hospital management team.

Go to www.dummies.com/extras/getintonursing schooluk for free online bonus content created especially for this book.

In this part . . .

- ✔ Chart your academic path to nursing school, from GCSEs to Access courses.
- ✔ Choose the best subjects to prepare you for nursing school.
- ✔ Polish your caring characteristics.
- ✔ Find help with dealing with health or learning issues.
- ✔ Gain care experience in a variety of settings.

Chapter 3

Weighing Academic Qualifications

• •

In This Chapter

▶ Understanding why academic qualifications are important

▶ Getting to grips with qualifications

▶ Finding out where you are and where you need to be

▶ Reviewing non-academic qualifications

• •

*M*any people have a vision of nurses working with patients and undertaking clinical activities, whether on a hospital ward, in the patient's own home or in a community setting. Few people imagine a nurse sitting in a library with their head in a book! However, education and learning play a significant part in your career as a nurse, and this chapter introduces you to the first part of life-long learning in nursing.

The Nursing and Midwifery Council (NMC) requires all nursing students to undertake a degree programme of study and go to university.

This chapter explains the usual academic qualifications needed by candidates to prepare for university. It helps you consider the most appropriate qualifications, or, if you've already achieved your qualifications, how they relate to the university requirements.

Don't be put off by the emphasis on academic qualifications in this chapter! While studying is important, when you get to nursing school, you spend an equal amount of time in clinical practice, working with qualified nurses delivering actual care to patients.

Recognising the importance of a degree

Although students have learnt relevant subjects such as anatomy and physiology for many years, it's only since the 1990s that all student nurses have received academic qualifications alongside their professional registration. Controversy still exists over the pros and cons of degree education for nurses, and you may question the need to undertake a high level of academic study to care for patients. Here are some reasons that help to explain the importance of having graduate nurses:

✔ Healthcare constantly evolves, and the treatment and care of patients is becoming more complex.

✔ Nursing needs to respond to the greater expectation of quality control and accountability to the public and organisations such as the Care Quality Commission in England.

✔ Future nursing practice will be more advanced, and higher levels of knowledge and skill are required.

Charting Your Academic Path

The NMC doesn't make any requirements upon the entry qualifications of nursing programmes other than to stipulate basic skills in numeracy, reading and writing and computer skills. Each university then interprets these requirements to set all other levels of qualifications for their particular nursing programmes, so you can expect a lot of variation.

You can apply to up to five different universities. Research your chosen universities, and find out what academic qualifications they expect, as they may all ask for different subjects or grades. Chapter 11 offers advice on how UCAS can help with your search, and visit the website or read the prospectus for each university you're interested in.

If you contact admission tutors to discuss how your qualifications match the entry criteria, have your certificates to hand. Knowing the awarding body, level of study and number of credits is useful information that the admissions tutor needs to advise you correctly. (I explain credits in the later section 'Getting the Points'.)

Still at school

The advantage if you're still at school is that you're studying the most up to date subjects and have easy access to advice and support.

Schools are proactive in helping you plan for higher education, and many have careers events so you can meet university admissions teams.

When planning your future learning consider the following:

✔ Ensure you have sufficient GCSEs in the right subjects and grades.

✔ Which subjects are your strongest and which can give you the best overall grades.

✔ Which subjects are better for nursing and whether some universities require specific subjects.

If you want to talk to someone other than your teachers or your school's careers team, contact Connexions, who offer impartial career advice to 13–19 year olds: `https://www2.cxdirect.com/home.htm`

Applicants with life experience

'Life experience' is the politically correct term for 'mature'! Returning to study to ensure you have the right qualifications for nursing requires a more focused level of planning. You may have been away from study for several years yet gained life experience that could contribute to your application such as managing money, writing reports or taking the lead on projects.

'Topping up' on qualifications already achieved is sometimes sufficient, or a complete programme of study may be required, especially if you left school as 16. Put your own plan together so you can focus on what you need to achieve, and consider the following:

✔ Consider the qualifications you already have and how they compare to the entry criteria.

✔ How much time and what finances you can dedicate to learning.

✔ Are you an independent learner or do you thrive on peer support?

Approach your local college of further education to find out the courses available to you that can give you the qualifications you need to get on to a nursing degree.

All qualifications are explained in terms of levels; the more difficult the study, the higher the level. For example, level 1 means achieving GCSEs with grades D–G, whereas in level 8 work you'd be achieving a doctorate. To get into nursing school concentrate on levels 2 and 3:

- ✔ **Level 2:** Sometimes known as *intermediate level* courses, these are the foundation qualifications that universities expect you to have to demonstrate a range of general knowledge. Examples of these courses are:
  - GCSE subject with grades A*–C
  - BTEC First Diploma
- ✔ **Level 3:** Also known as *advanced level,* these are qualifications that often develop from level 2 subjects. The depth of study and assessment of knowledge are that much greater. Examples are:
  - Access courses
  - AS and A-levels
  - BTEC National Diploma

I explain these in more detail in the relevant sections later in the chapter. (Note: Scotland has a different system.)

Many nursing schools hold open days so you can meet with lecturers and discuss your aspirations. Some local authorities offer advice on further education. Search for your local Connexions (which also offers advice for adults), via a search engine or Yellow Pages. Alternatively, Learndirect is a useful starting point (www.learndirect.co.uk) for beginning your nursing studies.

Why Currency Counts: Assessing Your Study Skills

No, I'm not talking about sterling and euros here; *currency* means the *age* of your qualification and your *ability* to study as a student.

If you're returning to learning, you may have been told that the 'shelf life' of your qualification has expired and you can't use it towards going to university. This doesn't mean your qualification is now worthless; you worked hard and demonstrated your academic development over a period of time. You just need to refresh your qualification.

The length of time since achieving a qualification has a significant impact on your application to nursing school for two specific reasons:

✔ **Your study skills.** You should have undertaken study in the last three to five years to demonstrate your skills are still fresh. These skills are about your ability to manage the rigours of higher education and include using the library, searching online databases, preparing for lectures, writing academic essays and managing submission dates. Nursing students work a significantly longer academic year than other university students and admission tutors want to make sure that candidates have a smooth transition to university study – you will of course have help and advice on the programme!

Some universities accept work-based skills as a way of demonstrating study skills. Depending on your career to date, you may already have appropriate evidence; skills such as ability to write reports, maintain schedules or deliver presentations could all be useful.

✔ **The content and grade of your qualification.** Course material and assessment methods can alter to reflect the changing employment market. The subjects you studied many years ago and the way you were assessed may no longer meet the requirements for today's degree programmes. For example an O-level in biology gained 15 years ago sadly is of little help in how you're taught and assessed on human physiology today!

Resit, or move on?

Admissions tutors are compassionate souls (honest) and are willing to offer reasonable support to a candidate's aspirations to become a nurse. But the demands of higher education do require a realistic approach to selection, and admission tutors choose those candidates who show the best potential (academically and professionally) to be successful on the degree programme.

If you fail to achieve the grade you need to get on a nursing course, think about the merits of re-sitting the qualification. Moving from a D grade to a C grade may require only a small movement in assessment scores, whereas trying to retrieve an E grade would require a significant improvement in your understanding and ability in the subject.

Nursing programmes have intensive periods of study that often coincide with clinical placements. Admissions tutors are looking for candidates who demonstrate the ability to study many subjects consecutively.

Admissions tutors can be sceptical of course changes as it can indicate that the student is struggling with the teaching and learning methods and is desperate to find a course that suits them. Be prepared to explain why you changed courses and how your new course better prepares you for university.

If you're like me, you stashed away your academic certificates in a box up in the attic. You need to climb up there, hunt them out and dust them down. Having your certificates in front of you helps you compare them against what is currently asked for, and also having all the information in front of you makes it much easier if you need to contact the admissions tutor.

Back to Basics: GCSEs

Many universities require you to have a good GCSE profile that includes a number of subjects with grades between A and C. The most common core subjects are English language, maths and science. Often, even when you've undertaken higher qualifications such as A-levels, not having the right GCSEs can cause problems for your application.

If you're considering GCSEs (General Certificate of Secondary Education) at the same time as applying for nursing, you most likely left school with few GCSEs, studied outside the UK or are resitting some subjects. In these situations, consider:

- ✔ Do I have the core subjects needed for university?

- ✔ How many GCSEs are the universities expecting me to achieve?

- ✔ Do the universities expect a particular grade for some subjects?

GCSEs are traditionally studied over two years in school, but you can complete them in one year in further education colleges.

If you're a life experience student, you can pick and choose individual subjects relevant to your need rather than having to study set subjects as you do in school.

The NMC requires that nursing candidates demonstrate numeracy skills, abilities in reading and comprehension and computer skills. These are core skills and the requirements are interpreted by universities as GCSE level and are included in any entry requirement. GCSEs are graded from A* to G and U (unclassified). Universities only recognise grades A* to C as counting towards the entry criteria.

If you haven't achieved the core qualifications, some universities consider alternatives; for example, a university may consider Fundamental or Essential Skills Level 2 or 3 in numeracy instead of maths GCSE.

You can study GCSEs at two levels: the higher level is graded from A* to D, whereas the lower level is graded C to G. If you study at the lower level this restricts your top grade to C, which may not be good enough for some universities. How well you perform on the GCSE course determines the level you're assessed at and your course tutor can explain which level can give your best grade.

If the university wants to include GCSEs as part of their entry criteria, they often explain it in their UCAS profile. Here's an example:

> '5 GCSEs at grade C including maths, English and science. Functional skills in numeracy and literacy are accepted as alternatives. GCSE ICT is also desirable.'

Getting the Points

Once you start to plan your application it becomes clear very quickly that universities ask for different qualifications, despite the nursing programme outcomes being very much the same across the country. With so many qualifications to choose from and with each university asking for different grades it can all become very confusing.

But help is at hand. To unravel the confusion, UCAS attach points to each grade and each qualification. This helps you understand how your qualifications compare with other qualifications and how your grade corresponds to other grades. Universities use this system to ensure that all candidates have undertaken the same breadth and depth of learning regardless of which qualifications they have studied.

Here's an example of how each of these single subjects (say, biology) have similar points attached to them indicating the depth of knowledge needed for each qualification.

Biology A-level	A*	A	C	E
Biology BTEC	D*	D	M	P
UCAS Points	140	120	80	40

In this example I show the comparison for different grades for a full set of qualifications, which you're likely to need for university.

	A-level	*BTEC Extended Diploma*
Grades	BBC	Distinction Merit Merit
UCAS Points	280	280
Grades	CCC	Merit Merit Merit
UCAS Points	240	240

So the first thing to look for when applying for nursing school is how many points the university needs you to achieve. You can find this statement in the university's prospectus or on their UCAS profile. The statement can also tell you the level of study required to achieve the points; for example:

'280 UCAS tariff points with a minimum of 180 points required with the volume and depth of A-level or equivalent.'

This means:

✔ You must achieve 280 points overall.

✔ At least 180 of these points must come from A-levels or equivalents (such as BTEC).

✔ 100 points may come from qualifications lower than A-level (such as AS-level; GCSEs aren't considered in this type of offer).

Each university profile explains which qualifications are acceptable and any specific criteria for the qualification such as subject or grade.

You can only use points once for the same subject. You can't, for example, use points from both AS-level and A-level in biology. Only the higher level points count.

Aiming for A-levels (Advanced General Certificate of Education)

A-levels are recognised as the traditional entry requirements for most higher education courses and are the standard by which all other equivalent qualifications are compared. They're the principle examination courses for students after completing compulsory education and who are normally between the ages of 17 and 18. A-levels are traditionally taught over two years in school sixth forms or FE colleges where adult learners can also undertake the qualifications.

A-levels consist of two elements:

- **Advanced subsidiary level (AS).** Students can exit the first year with an AS award. Often seen as half an A-level, they carry 50 per cent of the points of an A-level. All students take the AS exams at the end of the first year of study; some accept the qualification, while others pursue the full A-level award next year. Students often take AS subjects alongside their chosen A-level subjects to demonstrate a broad range of learning.

- **Advanced level (A2).** Students who continue their studies study to full A-level for the second year and can achieve the Advanced GCE award. This award develops from and is more demanding than the AS qualification and carries the maximum number of UCAS points for the grades.

A-levels are assessed through formal examination and coursework, so expect to have to write essays, deliver presentations, complete reports and sit exams. Both AS and A-level awards are graded A* to E with U being an unclassified (fail) grade.

If you're still at school, A-levels are a great option for you. Picking appropriate subjects and getting good grades makes you a very strong candidate for nursing school.

As a life experience student, undertaking an A-level to demonstrate return to studying is a good option; but if you're using this qualification to gain all the entry criteria, you could find it very hard work. Mature students typically study A-levels full-time over one year, and attempting three A-levels could impact on your grades. Other options are BTEC and Access courses (covered later in this chapter).

Choosing your subjects

You have a wide variety of A-level subjects to choose from, and universities are flexible in which subjects they accept for nursing courses.

When choosing your subjects, check:

- **That your chosen university accepts all A-level subjects.** Some universities don't recognise particular subjects including General Studies and Critical Thinking.

- **For any special subject requirements.** Some universities ask for specific subjects at A-level and won't consider your application without them. Biology is a popular required subject.

✔ **If the university of your choice favours particular subjects.** Often universities suggest that certain 'health related' subjects would be an advantage to students. This means having the subject improves your chances of being chosen. Subjects such as sociology and psychology are often included as desirable subjects.

Think about how your choice of subjects demonstrates your commitment to nursing and accentuate this on your personal statement (Chapter 12 covers completing your personal statement). Universities look at your subjects to help determine whether you can cope with the academic study on the nursing degree. Some subjects have a clear assessment strategy of using essay and exams that make you a stronger candidate, such as maths, biology, English literature, law and geography.

Subjects that are less appealing to admissions tutors because they may not contain the type of studying or assessment that offers the best preparation for a nursing degree include ICT, media studies and art.

Some schools and colleges offer 'Health Sciences' courses. These courses contain many of the elements taught on nursing courses at university such as anatomy and physiology, psychology and sociology. These are appropriate subjects to choose and give you insight into teaching on nursing degrees.

Getting the grades

Universities ask for the level of qualification by grades or points. If they ask for grades, A* to C is the standard; if they ask for points, you can sometimes use grades D and E.

Not all universities allow AS grades to be used as part of your entry criteria. Those that do often stipulate the number of AS subjects allowed or limit the amount of UCAS points that you can use from AS grades.

Chapter 11 explains the UCAS process in detail, but here are examples of typical offers:

Grades: 'ABB, excluding General Studies and Critical Thinking.'

AS/A2: '280 points with a minimum of 2 A-levels at C grade and 3 AS-levels at C grade.'

Range: 'ACE, ADD, BCE, CCC, CCD.'

Getting Down to Business with BTECs

A BTEC (Business and Technology Education Council award) is a vocational qualification with an emphasis on employment.

Taught mostly in FE colleges full-time, part-time or by distance learning, many of the courses require you to spend a period of time in the relevant workplace.

BTECs are offered at many levels broadly equivalent to GCSEs through to degree level. For the purposes of university entry you need the level 3 National Diploma courses as a minimum. Titles such as *Certificate, Diploma* and *Extended Diploma* are good indicators of the right level. As always, check with your preferred nursing school about their requirements before embarking on a BTEC course.

With the focus on skills needed by employers, BTECs use a practical approach to assessments which are often combined with workplace commitments. Students complete a number of units to achieve the overall qualification; each unit is assessed by providing evidence based on actual work or studies, which could be an exam, task, test or a performance, depending on the subject. Progress is measured throughout the course and this type of ongoing assessment is great if you dislike end-of-year assessments.

Choosing your subjects

As the intention of BTECs is to offer real world experiences alongside academic study, the subjects relate closely to workplace roles. BTECs in Health and Social Care or Health Studies are the most appropriate for prospective nursing students as the focus is very much about society, health and care delivery.

Another preference is science-based subjects, because they help develop skills of applying knowledge to practical problems.

Level 3 courses are offered in different sizes depending upon the number of units studied, and this is broadly similar to choosing one, two or three A-levels. You usually study a full 18-credit course that's equivalent to three A-levels, but a popular alternative is to study two smaller courses that add up to the same larger qualification. This 'mix and match' approach means you can study two subjects, such as Applied Science and Health and Social Care.

Is a BTEC award a useful qualification for nursing?

BTECs are a very popular alternative to A-level qualifications, and many BTEC students are very successful on nursing programmes. The continual assessment methods of BTEC courses suit many candidates and are similar to some of the assessments in nursing. However you sit exams, write lengthy essays and pass assessments with few attempts at nursing school, which are not always covered on BTEC courses.

Some universities ask for a higher level of award for BTECs than they do for other qualifications, so the grades required may not match the points system. Check with the nursing school you want to attend before you apply.

Getting the grades

You're given an overall grade for the amount of units you studied, so you can achieve one, two or three grades depending on the size of the course. Each course is graded by name (Pass, Merit, Distinction) rather than by letter (like A-levels).

Two typical offer examples are:

> Grades only: 'Distinction, Distinction, Merit.'
>
> Grades and subjects: 'Merit, Merit, Merit. Health and Social Care or Applied Sciences preferred.'

Scottish Qualifications

Scotland uses a different system of qualifications than the rest of the UK. The Scottish Qualifications Authority (SQA) is responsible for the development and certification of Scottish qualifications.

At the lower levels students undertake *Standard Grades* that are broadly comparable to GCSE qualifications.

For purpose of applying to university you need to study at the *Higher* and *Advanced Higher* levels. These levels are assessed through coursework and normally an external examination. Grades are awarded ranging from A to D, but for university only grades A, B and C are considered.

The SQA emphasises the importance of core skills, which are luckily an essential part of the entry requirements for nursing and include:

- ✔ Numeracy
- ✔ Communication
- ✔ Problem solving
- ✔ Working with others
- ✔ Information technology

The SQA offers a wide range of subjects from arts and languages to physical and social sciences, and you can choose a range of subjects to demonstrate your breadth of study.

Typical offer examples are:

Higher Level: 'BBCC, AABBB – ABBBB, 240 points with a minimum of A grade in a science subject'

Advanced Higher: 'CC, AB, a minimum of 3 grades with at least a C grade in science.'

Talking About Access

Access to Higher Education courses are designed for students who want to undertake a university course but didn't gain the qualifications needed when at school. Originally Access courses were intended for the mature person returning to study, but today they're available to 18- to 19-year-olds as well. A feature of these courses is that the student has sufficient life experience to be able to cope with the demands of the study.

A popular alternative is for candidates to undertake a Pre-Access course before embarking on the full course, but this can add a few extra months onto the time you study at college before starting your nursing degree.

An Access course is designed for students with little or no formal academic qualifications, and so the assessments cover the equivalent of GSCE and A-level requirements. Taught through a series of units, you're assessed through a range of methods including exams, tests, essays and projects. Each unit is allocated a number of credits depending on the amount of study time needed to complete the unit.

There are two levels of assessment with the GCSE equivalents assessed at level 2 and A-level equivalents assessed at level 3. To pass the course you need to achieve 60 credits with a maximum of 15 from level 2 assessments and a minimum of 45 level 3 assessments.

Check out your local college of further education for details of Access courses or do some research online for distance learning.

Choosing your subjects

Access courses are designed with a specific university course in mind, and the subjects on the course reflect those delivered at university. Unsurprisingly, admission tutors expect nursing students to complete an Access course developed for entry into nursing. Courses with titles such as *Access to Nursing, Health Studies* or *Health Professions* are common, and science courses are also relevant.

Courses have mandatory and optional subjects. The optional subjects are useful if you're applying to numerous universities who all ask for slightly different subjects.

Getting the grades

You need to achieve Level 2 credits in numeracy and literacy even though they aren't graded. Level 3 credits are graded as *Pass, Merit* and *Distinction,* and you accumulate them as each unit is assessed. You don't get an overall grade award but a collection of grades.

Many universities don't consider applicants who simply pass their Access course, but require candidates to gain a number of merit or distinction grades too.

Typical offer examples are:

Type of course: 'Successful completion of Health and Social Care or Nursing course. 45 credits must be gained at Level 3 with 30 credits at Merit.'

Specific units required: 'Achieve Access Diploma. 15 credits at level 3 must be in biology and must be at merit grade.'

Specific grades: 'Achieve Access Diploma with a minimum profile of 6 Pass, 33 Merit and 6 Distinction grades.'

Access courses don't carry UCAS tariff points and you can't match grades against UCAS equivalents. Offers made by universities are against the grades and credits achieved on the course and not against UCAS points.

Is Access suitable for me?

Access has become a very popular course and of all the Access qualifications available, those used for entry to nursing are the most popular. If you're returning to study and have few qualifications, then Access can be a very good way of achieving the recognised entry qualifications.

If you already have good qualifications and just need to refresh your study skills, Access may be more intense than you actually need; a less demanding course may be suitable for your purposes.

 As Access courses are specifically designed for you to gain entry to university, all the students on the entry to nursing courses want to become – surprise, surprise – nurses or other healthcare professionals, so there's often a great camaraderie and peer support. However, just because the course is called 'Access to Nursing' doesn't mean you'll have a given right to gain entry to university!

Mixing 'n' matching qualifications

Perhaps you have many qualifications from various routes and your academic profile doesn't fit neatly into any category. Not to worry; universities can account for your collection of qualifications.

You can match up different qualifications to meet the entry criteria for nursing. Each qualification has its allocated points, and universities can tell you if you can use them as part of your profile.

However, Access is the exception to this rule because it's a purpose built course designed to give all the necessary entry requirements in a single qualification, so you can't add parts of it to other qualifications.

Combination examples include:

✔ Welsh Baccalaureate *plus* 2 A-levels

✔ BTEC National Diploma *plus* 1 A-level

✔ Two A-levels *plus* BTEC Subsidiary Diploma

Not all qualifications are accepted by universities. It is quite normal to see *not accepted* written alongside some qualifications, and this indicates you cannot use the qualification as evidence that you meet the entry requirements.

(continued)

(continued)

Some of the more unusual qualifications that have been accepted for nursing programmes include:

✔ AAT Level 3 Diploma in Accounting

✔ CACHE Award in Child Care and Education

✔ Certificate in Financial Services

✔ Level 3 Award in Community Volunteering

And here are some that haven't:

✔ British Horse Society Awards

✔ Music/Rockschool Awards

✔ Certificate of Personal Effectiveness

✔ Diploma in Fashion Retail

Check all of your qualifications against the entry profile for each of the universities that interest you. Your qualification may be accepted by one university and not another.

Certificates, Foundation and University Degrees

Certificates, foundation and university degrees are delivered at a higher educational level than A-levels and exceed any UCAS point requirements set by the universities. All of these qualifications are very academically focused and follow traditional learning and assessment methods. Expect to spend time in the classroom and a considerable amount of time with self-directed study. You're usually assessed through exams, tests, essay and projects.

Certificate and foundation qualifications are becoming more popular for students who didn't achieve the grades or points needed at A-level standard but prefer a higher level of study – or people returning to study who don't want to repeat A-levels. Many of these qualifications have a healthcare focus and have modules appropriate to nursing:

✔ *Certificate* level courses are usually equivalent to the first year of university. These courses are tailored to help you get onto your career pathway and so a Certificate to Health Studies or Science would be most suitable. These courses are built up of a number of modules, which you will be expected to pass to complete the course.

✔ *Foundation degrees* are often used for people who want a qualification related to their work but don't want the full professional qualification; a good example of this is a foundation degree in dental nursing. These qualifications are equivalent to two years at university level and are very good at linking a higher level of study with employment skills.

Choosing a course that's health or science focused makes your application stronger, especially if you don't have top A-level grades.

Perhaps you have a degree already, but in a subject not related to nursing. This demonstrates your ability to study at a higher level but you also need to show how the study has prepared you for the nursing programme.

Many students who have a first degree before starting nursing comment on how different the courses are. Due to the long academic year and clinical placements, graduates can take just as long to settle into nursing courses as those without degree experience.

Although all of the courses are at a high academic level, make sure you meet the minimum requirements for numeracy, as some universities won't consider you without your GCSE in maths.

If you have a good classification in an honours degree that's relevant to healthcare, a two-year master's nursing programme could be a very good option for you. Take a look at your preferred universities to see if they offer this option.

The flexible approach: The Open University

The Open University (OU) has a world-class reputation for delivering education through distance learning. The option of studying in your spare time is becoming more popular as students have to balance work and life commitments. While the Open University offers a nursing programme, it has some restrictions such as having to be sponsored by your employer, which prevents many candidates from applying.

The OU is becoming very popular as a means of gaining entry qualifications to other universities. Many mature students find taking some of the level 1 modules to be an ideal way of updating their study skills and filling the gaps in their educational profile.

If you're unable to study full-time or can't commit to set study hours each week, enrolling with the OU could be a good option. Consider the health and social care modules and work towards achieving a minimum of 60 credits (such as the Introduction to Health Care module).

OU modules can be expensive: do your research and check that your chosen universities accept OU modules, and find out which subjects they prefer.

Tasting the Fruit of Experience: APEL

Universities strive to ensure that they recruit the best candidates to their courses and understand that sometimes these candidates don't follow a typical educational route. Experienced students may have missed opportunities for higher education when they were younger or followed a different career, but now aspire to a change of career direction. Perhaps you feel you already have much to offer nursing, for example you may have run your own business and have valuable experience in teamwork, managing deadlines, numeracy skills and managing priorities.

Accreditation of Prior and Experiential Learning (APEL) is a process that enables you to receive formal recognition for skills and knowledge you already possess. This process is used to:

- ✔ Gain entry onto the nursing programme.

- ✔ Give exemption from certain parts of the nursing programme.

- ✔ Qualify for an award against an appropriate nursing subject.

The APEL process takes into account any organised prior learning where you've been formally assessed and awarded a qualification. Unstructured learning experiences such as short courses and work-based learning may count too.

If you want to use APEL to get into nursing school, you need to provide in-depth evidence of your learning experiences and map these against the nursing programme. This is a lengthy process and requires a great deal of information gathering, but it can result in having significant portions of the nursing programme excluded. Examples where this could be useful are:

- ✔ An applicant who qualified as a nurse in another country, but their registration is not currently recognised by the NMC.

- ✔ A support worker who uses clinical experience and study to be exempt from the first year.

- ✔ An ex-army medic who uses on-the-job experiences to be exempt from emergency care modules.

 The APEL process takes time, energy and money. Gathering all your evidence into a portfolio before approaching the university can greatly improve the advice they can offer. Each university has its own APEL process, and based on your portfolio can tell you how much work is needed to assess your experiences and how much money it'll cost you to have the assessments completed.

Using Foreign Qualifications

You may have undertaken your exams abroad and hope to use them against the university entry criteria. This is quite acceptable, but the process can be a little more complicated than using UK qualifications. While admissions tutors have some understanding of foreign qualifications, they won't know the precise details and comparison tariffs of them all.

Nailing the lingo

The NMC require all nursing students to be able to communicate effectively with other healthcare professionals, members of the public, and patients and their carers in English. You need to be able to talk, read and write to a standard that's clear and understandable to others.

As part of the selection procedure when you apply for nursing school, the admissions team assess you against the following criteria:

✔ How you manage to listen to conversations and respond in an appropriate manner to demonstrate your understanding of what's been said.

✔ Following written instructions or interpreting graphs and illustrations in PowerPoint or on handouts.

✔ Written tests or completion of paperwork, forms and documents.

✔ Answering questions in an interview, group work or during discussion sessions.

Most UK-taught students use the GCSE English language qualification to demonstrate these skills and need a C grade or above. Some universities accept equivalent essential skills in English or a communication subject.

For international students or candidates whose first language isn't English, two qualifications are generally used to assess English language skills. You need to complete one of these tests if you haven't undertaken a course of study in the UK:

✔ *The International English Language Testing System (IELTS)*. This system tests and scores your reading, writing, listening and speaking abilities. For nursing you undertake the academic-level test and need to achieve a minimum score of 7 for each of the four categories. Visit www.ielts.org/default.aspx.

✔ *Test of English as a Foreign Language system (TOEFL)*. You're assessed and scored in reading, writing, listening and speaking. Each domain has a maximum score of 30, and you typically need to achieve an overall score of 110. See www.ets.org/toefl.

UK NARIC (National Recognition Information Centre) is the UK's national agency responsible for providing comparison information for academic qualifications from across the world. It's managed on behalf of the UK government and is the only official source of educational qualifications attained outside of the UK.

You need to make an application to UK NARIC who, for the relevant fee, can produce a statement of comparison, which you can use as part of your application. Having this information helps you decide if you can apply for nursing immediately or undertake further study to meet the entry requirements.

You can find information about UK NARIC, its services and fees, at www.ecctis.co.uk/naric/.

Chapter 4

Professional Requirements: How Do You Rate?

*H*ow would you react if the nurse taking your blood pressure was struggling to examine you properly and smelled of alcohol? What would you do if you read in the local newspaper that the nurse caring for your young child had been cautioned for using abusive language to a police officer? Would it concern you that the nurse taking your details kept writing down the wrong information?

Nurses are ordinary people, live ordinary lives and have the same problems as everyone else. You can expect that occasionally nurses get themselves into trouble, become ill or suffer a life-changing event. What you don't expect, however, is that when life throws up challenges, nurses deliver substandard care, put their patients at risk or bring the profession into disrepute. For a nurse, professionalism is key.

In this chapter I explain what professional regulation means to potential student nurses. I introduce you to the concept of good health and good character, and why appreciating your social and professional responsibilities is important. Nurses have to be fit to practise and conduct themselves with extraordinary vigilance, and this chapter puts into context the reasons that your application for a nursing programme places so much emphasis on your attitude, behaviour and abilities. Use this chapter to check that you have what it takes to be professional as a nurse.

Reviewing Your Fitness to Practise

Nursing is a *self-regulating profession*, which means that it monitors the competence, attitude and behaviour of its members. The Nursing and Midwifery Council (NMC) has the legislative power to investigate and serve judgement on qualified nurses who fall below acceptable standards. The NMC also sets the standards for the education and training of student nurses and instructs universities in the way they recruit candidates and review student progress.

The NMC use the term *fitness to practise* to illustrate that nurses need to be capable of giving safe and effective care without supervision when they're qualified. Universities also look for fitness to practise when reviewing applicants who want to become a student nurse, looking for good character and good health in four areas:

- ✔ Monitoring your professional behaviour.

- ✔ Checking your criminal history.

- ✔ Reviewing your health and wellbeing.

- ✔ Taking into consideration any disabilities.

All universities have a *Fitness to Practise Committee* that reviews the evidence available on these four elements and decides whether you can proceed onto the nursing programme or not. The committee normally consists of a senior university manager, admission tutors, members of the Disability and Occupational Health Team, a senior nurse and a legal representative. The committee ensures that your application is considered fairly and with appropriate attention to professional standards.

When it comes to the health and disability criteria, the committee can't apply a set formula to all candidates, so it starts from the point that with reasonable adjustment all applicants are suitable for the programme. Reasonable adjustment recognises the need to follow The Equality Act 2010 Codes of Practice that expect assessments to focus on what adjustments are acceptable to help you gain a place and be successful on the programme. Reasonable adjustment doesn't change the outcomes of the programme, so although you may have help and assistance during your training, you have to achieve the same outcomes to register as a nurse as everyone else.

The university treats each application individually, and only if adjustments become unreasonable would you become aware that your application has been reviewed by the committee. This committee business sounds very ominous, but in reality the majority of applicants who have an offer of a place find their application runs smoothly.

The following sections look at each of the four areas under review by the committee in turn, and show you how to make sure your application ticks the right boxes.

Monitoring Your Professional Behaviour

Becoming a professional requires insight into what is expected of the profession, not only by the regulating body (the NMC) but also by the university and members of the public. Chapter 5 gives more detail on how you're expected to behave, but here I briefly list some instances where the Fitness to Practise Committee would question your good character:

- ✔ Not confirming attendance or arriving late to a selection event.
- ✔ Having poor attendance at college or work.
- ✔ Having your personal statement reported for plagiarism.
- ✔ Hounding the university for updates on your application.
- ✔ Making derogatory comments about others on social networks.
- ✔ Showing lack of respect to administrative staff.

 You're being assessed for your professional behaviour as soon as you engage in the application process. You want to be known to the admissions tutor for all the *right* reasons.

 If you want to know how the NMC expects you to behave, have a read of their guidance on professional conduct for student nurses at www.nmc-uk.org/Students/Guidance-for-students.

'Ello, 'Ello: Examining Your Criminal Record

Having a criminal record is quite an emotive subject that causes a great amount of anxiety for nursing candidates. Universities don't set out to bar candidates with a criminal history from nursing, but they must ensure that nursing students pose no risk to patients and the public. From this viewpoint, you can see that minor infringements, such as reprimands or cautions, don't cause any serious problems to your application, whereas a conviction with a lengthy custodial sentence is likely to prevent you gaining a nursing offer.

Universities check the criminal history of each applicant and make decisions against the background checks. Policies differ slightly between universities, but you're not allowed to attend clinical practice until a check has been performed and a decision made about your suitability to nurse.

Government organisations carry out the checks. They review all the information held on you by the police and other enforcement agencies. Until recently the Criminal Records Bureau checked for criminal history and the Independent Safeguarding Agency checked whether you're barred from working with children or vulnerable adults. In 2012 these two agencies merged into the Disclosure and Barring Service (DBS).

Early disclosure is the best tactic to reduce stress and, you have three opportunities to do this:

- **Before applying:** Some universities may ask you to provide more information at the point of application about your criminal record. Contact the university for advice on their policy and how it affects your application. If you have a criminal record, you may find out straight away that the seriousness of your conviction is such that you will not be accepted.

- **UCAS application:** The application form asks whether you have any relevant criminal history. If you have a criminal record, no matter how insignificant you believe it to be, then answer positively.

- **University selection process:** Interviewers ask about your criminal record as a way of double-checking your understanding of the UCAS question. The interviewer isn't there to pass judgement, so if you have a record, simply state the type of offence, the year it happened and some basic facts.

You may have been given advice that you don't have to disclose your caution or conviction. The Rehabilitation of Offenders Act 1974 allows for criminal convictions to be declared 'spent' after a period of time, so in normal circumstances you don't have to disclose those convictions. But nursing is exempt from the Act and applicants must always disclose their full criminal history.

When reviewing your record the university is looking for cautions or convictions that may be incompatible with professional registration. It considers the following issues:

✔ Whether you disclosed the caution or conviction.

✔ The length of time since the offence and nursing application.

✔ Any pattern of re-offending.

✔ The circumstances surrounding the offence and your explanation of the offence.

✔ Your commitment to work safely and effectively, upholding the trust and confidence of patients and clients.

✔ The degree of risk you pose to patients and clients.

Infractions you can live with

Minor driving offences such as speeding fines don't appear on your criminal record. Minor infringements of the law, such as cautions for being drunk and disorderly or petty theft, will probably be acceptable as long as you disclose them, and you may not have to attend a meeting to discuss these.

Universities undertake an *enhanced* criminal record check. This includes all records that would normally be classed as spent. Should even minor infringements appear on your record that you hadn't disclosed then you'd be required to explain why.

Take this example: Julie is a 34-year-old mother. Once, when 16 and still at school, she was pressured into shoplifting with some girls from school. She was caught and cautioned at the police station. On applying for adult nursing, Julie forgets all about this caution – the only mark on her criminal record – and doesn't disclose it. She is shocked to be called to an exploratory meeting to discuss her non-disclosure. She shows remorse and the panel agrees that Julie is no risk to patients and is now of good character, so they uphold the decision to offer her place. Julie is lucky – failing to disclose her full criminal record had counted against her application.

Convictions incompatible with nursing

If you've been convicted of a serious offence then expect to be rejected for nursing regardless of the time and circumstances of the offence. Such offences include:

✔ Child abuse and abuse of vulnerable adults.

✔ Dealing in drugs.

✔ Entry on any of the protection lists with the Disclosure and Barring Service.

✔ Grievous bodily harm.

✔ Sex abuse and sexual offences.

Many offences are borderline cases and the decision to accept or decline your application can often hinge on how you present your case. Expect to attend an exploratory meeting if you have reprimands, cautions or convictions for offences such as common assault and battery, drug offences, antisocial behaviour, drunk driving or offences that show lack of honesty or trustworthiness such as fraud and theft. You need to discuss the issues in a frank and forthright manner that demonstrates you have moved forward since the offence, you appreciate the seriousness of having a positive record and you understand how it affects being a professional nurse.

Here are two examples of applicants with convictions that are red flags for universities:

✔ **The accepted applicant:** In his teenage years, John was convicted of drunk driving and banned for 12 months. At the exploratory meeting John explains the circumstances surrounding his conviction, his remorse and how he has moved on in the past four years: he is now teetotal, working part-time as a volunteer and is passionate about becoming a mental health nurse. The panel decides John is of good character and of no risk to patients, and his offer of a nursing place is upheld.

✔ **The rejected applicant:** Charlotte is a mature student who wants to be a children's nurse. Two years ago she was cautioned for antisocial behaviour and common assault. At her exploratory interview, she explains that both offences were against a woman who showed interest in her boyfriend. She becomes agitated as she explains the events, and declares that while fighting is not the best way to settle a problem, it is her right to protect her self-respect. Charlotte's application is denied, because the panel feels that she has little perspective on how nurses are expected to behave, she shows no remorse for her actions and she doesn't demonstrate the level of self-awareness expected from student nurses.

Taking Health and Wellbeing into Consideration

To deliver safe and effective nursing care, you need to be in good health. This is for the benefit of both you and the patients:

✔ **Patients:** Nurses can't place patients at risk because of their own health conditions. For example, you can't expose your patient to harmful infections, and neither can your mental health cause you to be neglectful when performing your duties.

✔ **You:** Nursing is demanding, not only intellectually but also physically and mentally. Even with all the aids and equipment available, the practical aspects of nursing require a level of physical stamina that can be too much for some students. In addition, if your health is poor, you should not be around infectious patients. And nursing has a high emotional toil, so candidates who suffer from mental health disorders may find they struggle to cope with the emotional demands of the course.

Having good health doesn't mean the absence of any physical or psychological conditions, but rather that these illnesses don't impair your ability to practise safely. Most people with long-term conditions are able to practise and meet the NMC expectations with no or little adjustment to their practice.

Unless you request otherwise, the Fitness to Practise Committee only reviews your health and wellbeing once you accept the offer of a place.

You have to comply with the healthcare provider's inoculation policies such as hepatitis B and tuberculosis screening. If you object to these on medical, ethical or personal grounds, discuss this with the admissions team.

You complete a health declaration form and sometimes meet with the Occupational Health Team. They discuss many aspects of your condition and make a decision as to whether you're fit for the programme and what, if any, adjustments need to be made.

Health issues and adjustments

No definitive list of ailments and conditions that are or are not acceptable exists, because needs are assessed individually; what's helpful for one student could be a hindrance to another. Here are some questions to ask yourself about your health and wellbeing to explore how you would cope on the programme:

✔ Do you make frequent visits to your GP or consultant, and how much time each month do you need for these?

✔ Are you able to undertake physical work for hours at a time without becoming exhausted?

✔ Do you need frequent rest breaks to take medicine or food and drinks?

✔ How do you cope in emotional situations, such as dealing with challenging behaviour? Do you become overly stressed and anxious about such incidences?

The university will consider adjusting parts of the programme to accommodate your health and wellbeing if necessary. For example, they may agree to rearrange your shifts to reduce the impact of long hours and unsocial shift patterns, or allow short rest breaks during exams.

Situations that present a challenge

If the adjustments needed to support you on the programme require significant investment, major changes to the programme or considerable support in clinical practice, the university may not support your application. In these situations the Fitness to Practise Committee will inform you of the decision, explain the reasons for the decision and offer advice on how you can move forward.

Consider this example. Dave has successfully applied for adult nursing, and after a good interview has been offered a place on the programme. But then Dave is diagnosed with bipolar disorder. The Fitness to Practise Committee decides that because Dave was currently receiving treatment for a newly diagnosed condition, for his own wellbeing it would be inappropriate to continue with the offer. The university encourages Dave to get in touch when his GP is confident that his condition is stable enough for him to resume his application.

Dealing with Disability

Universities comply with the Equality Act 2010 and will make all reasonable adjustments to support students with disabilities; they have a dedicated team of experienced staff who help assess your needs, support you in applying for funding and arrange for the pro-curement of equipment as necessary. These teams may also have experience of healthcare and clinical practice and are very suc-cessful in enabling students with particular needs to have a posi-tive experience at university.

When applying, UCAS gives you the choice to disclose any disability. You may be concerned that disclosing your disability at this stage disadvantages your application, but rest assured this isn't the case. The Fitness to Practise Committee, not the admissions tutors, make these decisions; early disclosure only speeds up receiving appropriate assessment and help.

Check out university websites to find out how they help their students with disabilities. These web pages contain very useful information on where, when and how to get support in readiness for you starting the programme.

Making every effort

The Equality Act 2010 defines that a person has a *disability* if they have a physical or mental impairment and the impairment has a substantial and long-term adverse effect on their ability to perform normal day-to-day activities. Obviously, this definition covers many conditions and illnesses, but depends upon the severity of the condition. A student nurse with asthma, for example, may have no problems coping with the day-to-day activities of student life, whereas a student with brittle asthma, which is difficult to control and causes frequent asthmatic attacks, requires considerable adjustments to their education.

Universities work closely with applicants to decide if they can be supported on the programme. To help your application, consider these tips:

- ✔ If you already have an assessment of your disabilities, keep the report handy to show the admissions team.

- ✔ Gain some experience of what nurses do in practice. Understanding how to cope with daily skills and activities is much easier when you have experienced them in a health setting rather than just read about them.

- ✔ Have a realistic understanding of what the programme outcomes entail. Find out what you need to do to pass the programme.

- ✔ You're the expert in knowing your disability: share your views so people can understand.

Coping with dyslexia

Of all disabilities dyslexia is the most common one in nursing. Ordinarily, this learning difficulty isn't an issue for the Fitness to Practise Committee if the student receives help and support. When concerns are raised, the team considers how dyslexia may cause problems with your safe and effective practice. Consider the characteristics below and how they might impact on your studies.

✓ **Memory difficulties:** Forgetting the names of patients, drugs or medical conditions; finding it difficult to learn routines and procedures.

✓ **Organisational difficulties:** Struggling to follow instructions correctly; reacting slowly in emergency situations.

✓ **Time management:** Submitting coursework late; struggling to balance coursework and practice commitments.

✓ **Reading and language:** Struggling to read handwritten text in noisy environments; being unable to express yourself with the right words.

✓ **Writing and spelling:** Needing extra time to fill out forms and reports; Mixing up letters and numbers.

✓ **Motor skills:** Having difficulty following sequences; struggling with left and right coordination.

The RCN has a helpful toolkit for dyslexia at www.rcn.org.uk/__data/assets/pdf_file/0003/333534/003835.pdf

An example: Hilary has applied for learning disability nursing. She's suffered from rheumatoid arthritis for the last six years and has several relapses every two to three months. On accepting the offer of a place on the nursing programme she completes the health and wellbeing form and attends a health check with an occupational health nurse. She's honest with the nurse about her condition – including details of stiffness in her wrist that makes writing difficult. The nurse writes a report for the Fitness to Practise Committee suggesting that Hilary is capable of undertaking the programme so long as during her relapses she is allowed to use a voice recorder for lessons rather than writing notes, with the lecturer and lecture group's consent. These adjustments were seen as reasonable and the offer of her place was upheld.

When adjustments just can't be made

A candidate with a realistic understanding of nursing usually appreciates early on in the application process whether their disability is of an extent that they'll have great difficulty achieving all the outcomes of the programme. But sometimes candidates aren't aware of these limitations and need supporting in a sensitive manner. The university keeps such applicants informed of decisions and their reasons, and often the admission team offers appropriate careers advice.

Julian has poor eyesight and hearing. The occupational health nurse refers him to the Fitness to Practise Committee. The committee decides that although Julian could use specialised equipment, he would struggle to develop many practical skills in assessing patients, reading notes, writing reports and planning care. Therefore, they decide that Julian would not be able to deliver safe and effective care even with the available adjustments and they decline to proceed with the offer of a place. A member of the panel met with Julian to offer advice, and subsequently he enrolled onto a medical sciences degree at the university, a pure academic programme that would lead to other opportunities of work in healthcare.

Plenty of advice is available to help you make the right decisions. These websites are good starting points: the National Bureau for Students with Disabilities (www.skill.org.uk) and Disability Toolkits (www.disabilitytoolkits.ac.uk/students).

Chapter 5

Proving Your People Skills

A s human beings we are driven to relate to each other, and being around people is an essential basic need. However, when someone is ill or vulnerable, these basic needs become amplified: the person needs to be reassured that he's safe and in good hands. A big part of a nurse's job is therefore providing reassurance.

This chapter is about those characteristics that offer reassurance and how they relate to your application to nursing. I explain what the admissions team are looking for in you and how they assess your range of people skills that demonstrate your potential to be a good student nurse.

As you read through this chapter, notice the overlapping themes, such as respect and attentiveness. Many aspects of people skills lend themselves to the concept of caring.

It's not only during the interview that the admissions team consider your suitability for nursing: many opportunities occur before, during and after the interview to help inform their decision. Think of your people skills in your overall performance in the application.

Understanding Nursing Behaviours and Values

Nursing care in the UK is evolving to ensure that the way nurses act continues to have a significant positive impact on the quality of care that people receive. This vision is to recognise the values and behaviours that encapsulate what those in the caring profession do. One of the roles of the admissions tutor is to ensure that you demonstrate those behaviours and values, and they use two main organisations as guidance.

Health boards

The UK has four *health boards*: one each for England, Northern Ireland, Scotland and Wales, and they're responsible for improving the health outcomes for people in your area. As part of their role, they work alongside your local healthcare team to ensure that all the services are of good quality. They've identified behaviours and values that contribute to high-quality and compassionate care:

- ✓ **Care.** Through their whole lives patients expect to receive care that's consistently of high quality. The nurse demonstrates care through clinical skills and also behaviour and attitude.

- ✓ **Compassion.** Developing relationships built on empathy, kindness, respect and dignity leads to compassionate care. Nurses are expected to demonstrate skills of delivering care that promotes trust and understanding with the patient.

- ✓ **Competence.** Nurses must have the knowledge, skills and attitude to provide good-quality care that's supported by the best available evidence. Having the capability to use research and evidence in care delivery is an important aspect of nursing.

- ✓ **Communication.** Having good communication skills is about appreciating the patient's view of his health problems and responding in a manner that reflects the patient's concerns and allows the patient to make decisions. Nurses should also demonstrate good inter-professional communication skills as well.

- ✓ **Courage.** In the context of nursing, courage relates to the ability to manage difficult situations and speak up when things are wrong, to ensure that patients receive the right care. This may involve reporting another practitioner to their mentor or a member of the hospital management team.

- ✓ **Commitment.** Nurses must see the job through to the end and take action to achieve the best possible outcomes for the patients and for nursing as a whole.

Policies and documents for the health boards of the UK may be called different things, but the themes are the same. I chose the Commission Board for England to illustrate the themes.

NMC

In their *Standards for Nurse Education*, the NMC directs universities to develop certain skills with their students. These *Essential Skills Clusters* are a set of actions that the student must be competent at in order to progress from one year to the next before finally qualifying as a nurse. In total, five clusters exist, but those pertinent to this chapter relate to care, compassion and communication.

For a first-year student the NMC expects demonstration of professional image, trust, respect, kindness and responsiveness. According to the NMC, the student nurse:

- Is able to engage with people and build caring professional relationships.
- Takes a person-centred, personalised approach to care.
- Is attentive and acts with kindness and sensitivity.
- Interacts with the person in a manner that's interpreted as warm, sensitive, kind and compassionate, making appropriate use of touch.

Considering Caring Characteristics

Caring is a difficult concept to define because it's subjective to each person's culture, education and experience. Without getting into a deep philosophical debate, someone who cares wants to influence other people's lives for the better.

When assessing your potential to care, the admissions team reviews your attitude and your behaviour towards caring. This section helps you explore your strengths and weaknesses in this area.

Assessing your attitude

Attitudes make you who you are and they're quite difficult to change in the short term. Attitudes are a relatively stable construct and they influence how you're perceived by other people.

Consider your attitude to religion, for example. You probably have some understanding about religion: you may have experienced worship, you possibly observe rituals or wear religious symbols, and you no doubt have some well-defined opinions. Through your actions and expressions, others understand your attitude towards religion.

You display caring in the same way. Being sensitive to the feelings of others, thoughtful of their concerns, helpful and always responding positively to the anxieties of people, shows a disposition to caring. Review your attitude towards caring against these indicators:

- ✔ **Patience** is about creating or maintaining a sense of stability and peacefulness through the consideration of others. Do you allow others to take time making decisions or do you rush to take over tasks when others are too slow? Can you tolerate others people's deliberations? Are you able to listen to other opinions even when they become wearisome?

- ✔ **Honesty** is about being fair and sincere in your actions and responses. Do you treat everyone with respect? Can you accept responsibility for your own actions? Are you considerate in how you offer advice to others?

- ✔ **Trust** allows others to place confidence in your integrity. Can you maintain the confidentiality of information? Are others able to approach you without fear of reprisal? Are you reliable in your actions?

- ✔ **Humility** is about showing selflessness and giving respect. Can you accept criticism or accept praise gracefully? Do you put the concerns of others before your own? Are you modest in your daily activities, or are you excessive in all that you do?

Your attitude shows through on your UCAS application and through the way you conduct the whole process of applying. For example, continuously ringing the admissions team to find out the progress of your application doesn't demonstrate patience. Having a reference from your course tutor that says you struggle to accept criticism doesn't demonstrate humility! The admissions tutor uses all opportunities to assess if you have the appropriate attitude for nursing.

Exploring your behaviour

Universities look for behaviours in nursing candidates and expect you to display helping characteristics. When observing your actions it should be clear to the admissions team that you have a positive attitude towards caring, as evidenced in your behaviour.

Here's a list of behaviours that indicate a caring nature:

- ✔ You're available to those in need. For example, you make yourself accessible to patients who want to talk.

✔ You participate in informal social interactions, such as talking or being with others when it is not a requirement. Spending time with quieter colleagues to ensure they're included in the group demonstrates your ability to feel for others.

✔ You're attentive to what others say. You listen and use non-verbal cues, like nodding and smiling, to reinforce that you're giving someone your attention.

✔ You try to connect with others by actively seeking opportunities to get to know them, showing a real interest in who they are and what they feel while maintaining professional boundaries.

✔ Despite how tiresome it may be to go that 'extra mile', you're willing to put effort, time and emotion into the support of others.

The admissions tutor asks for references from your course tutor but also from your place of work or someone who knows you. These references are used to help determine that you have the right behaviour for nursing. Consider how you behave in your everyday activities and what others might say about your disposition towards caring. Chapter 13 covers how to get a reference.

Showing Compassion

Compassion is one of the core characteristics of good nursing care. *Compassion* is a deliberate participation with other people's suffering that goes beyond just understanding their suffering to actual identification with how they feel. So in nursing, compassion means more than just going through the motions of nursing care, but really feeling for the patient and getting involved.

Compassion is an important aspect from the selectors' point of view. Consider these statements made by nurses and patients:

'Compassion is having empathetic awareness of someone else's distress and a strong desire to relieve it.'

'Compassion makes the difference between giving care and giving meaningful care.'

'A patient feels really cared for when we nurses are thoughtful in what we do and say, because when we are thoughtful, we pay attention to the little details, the details that make such a difference.'

Attempting to identify which nursing candidates have the potential to become compassionate nurses can be problematic, because they need to see past an act put on in an interview. Admissions tutors need clear evidence to draw upon to indicate that you have the correct qualities.

Here are examples of how to demonstrate your compassionate nature, especially at selection events:

- **Show respect to others.** You do this by showing regard to authority, for instance being polite to administrative staff at the selection events or treating other candidates as your equals.

- **Engage with people to develop relationships and allow for mutual understanding.** You may not agree with everything someone says, but you're able to work alongside those whose have opinions differ to your own.

- **Be attentive to other people's concerns and anxieties.** You may be anxious yourself, but showing concern for others and being sensitive to their worries gives the admission tutor an insight into your compassionate side.

- **Treat others with dignity.** For example, when you meet people from different walks of life with diverse cultures, ethnicities and religions, show kindness and sensitivity. Your awareness and approach to these individuals will give recognition of your compassionate nature.

Proving Your Commitment

Being committed to nursing is an important factor that admission tutors consider when reviewing your application. Demonstrating your commitment is important for the following reasons:

- Being committed means you'll strive to succeed even when faced with difficult times on the programme.

- Committed people enthuse others. Being someone who's not easily discouraged inspires confidence in others and helps support those less-motivated members of the team.

- Nursing is about being reflective and learning for the future. If you show commitment, your effort over a period of time will be rewarded and you'll develop good levels of professionalism.

Consider these two quotes from nurses:

'I work with patients over long periods of time, so being committed to them is important in order to help them achieve good health and wellbeing.'

'Commitment is staying power, passion, seeing things through, to the end. It requires strength of character and belief to keep going and not lose sight of what you hope to achieve.'

Nursing is a rewarding profession, but also a very tough one. Long hours, physical exhaustion and emotional stress are all recognised aspects. Although nursing students are shielded from the full impact of these, the course involves a significant amount of hard work.

Admission tutors look for signs in your application that you're committed for the long haul, that you understand what it means to be a student nurse and that you have the staying power to complete the student nurse programme. Competition for places is high, so you don't want your application to leave the admissions tutor thinking you may leave the programme prematurely.

Admission tutors assess your commitment in two ways:

- ✔ **Personal commitment.** Your obligation (usually self-imposed) to your own personal development.

- ✔ **Nursing commitment.** The extent to which you act in accordance with the professional values and principles of nursing. Although there is ambiguity about society's expectation of nurses, professional commitment is very much reflected in your social and private life.

You aren't expected at this point of your application to demonstrate commitment at the level of a professional nurse, but the admissions tutor expects tangible evidence that you have the right attitude when it comes to achieving goals, working through problems and working as part of a team.

Here are some examples of how you can show you have the right attitude towards committing to nursing:

- ✔ **Be a member of a team or group.** Teamwork is an essential ingredient to effective people skills.

- ✔ **Achieve a good attendance record at school or college.** High absence rates illustrate lack of determination and effort and little grit to achieve personal goals; don't give this image!

Is your personality a good fit for nursing?

Evidence suggests that the personality of the nurse is core to the good care of the patient. Great nurses have a number of personality characteristics. The more you have, the better the nurse.

Look carefully at the following list. Do you have the right attributes to make a good nurse? How can you demonstrate these to the admissions tutor?

✔ You're flexible in your approach to responsibilities. Good nurses adjust and adapt with regards to work and family pressures.

✔ You have an eye for detail and can organise yourself to maintain high standards of care.

✔ You have stamina, energy and enthusiasm.

✔ You have excellent problem-solving skills and can adjust actions and behaviours quickly to support ever-changing clinical situations.

✔ You're emotionally strong and have composure in difficult situations.

✔ You have a good sense of humour!

✔ **Demonstrate a thorough understanding of nursing and why you have chosen a particular field.** In doing so you indicate that you have serious intentions towards nursing.

✔ **Gain care experience if possible.** Although some universities don't require care experience, your approach to understanding the value of such experience and relating your people skills to nursing expectations tells the admissions team much about your positive approach to nursing. Chapter 6 looks at getting care experience.

Communicating Effectively

You're probably familiar with the term *communication skills,* and you probably understand how useful these are. But do you really consider their importance on a daily basis? You act differently when relaxed and calm than you do when under scrutiny, and these relaxed moments reveal much about the real you. Many opportunities arise during the application process that bring your communication skills to an admission tutor's attention. In this section I explore some of the ways in which you communicate during your application, so you can avoid pitfalls and impress the university.

Email etiquette

Email is part of daily life, and it has some very good points. Emails arrive nearly instantaneously, can be accessed almost anywhere and can incorporate not only text but also pictures, documents, links and much more. These benefits make email a popular method of communication, and both UCAS and universities encourage you to use email when applying for nursing.

Email often doesn't receive the respect it deserves, and many candidates show little understanding of the impression an email gives admission tutors of their writing skills, levels of courtesy and ability to present a good image. First impressions count significantly in how the admissions tutor perceives you as a suitable candidate.

Here are few top tips to help your application stand out for the right reasons:

- ✔ **Use a sensible email address.** Do you still use the account you opened when in school? It may have sounded fun at the time, but names like 'Fairytippytoes@woohoo.com' or 'sexyclaire123@crazyplace.com' don't give the right impression. Consider opening a new account with a formal address for your university correspondence.

- ✔ **Use the subject box.** In the subject box set the context of your email. 'Advice regarding GCSE Biology' tells the reader what the email is about. Don't leave the box empty, forcing the recipient to read through your email to find out why you sent it.

- ✔ **Strike the right tone.** Make your first email courteous and formal: so 'Dear Mr Evered' and 'Yours sincerely'. Subsequent emails can be less formal, but always polite, following the lead of the other person: 'Hello, Andrew' to open and then 'Best regards' to close. Don't be too personal or rude: 'Hi there', 'Fondly yours' and 'Bye now' are inappropriate.

- ✔ **Avoid emoticons and text talk.** Using text speak and emoticons and exaggerating words can be fun when emailing friends, but in an email to university they show your inability to understand the type of relationship between yourself and the reader. 'Thanx 4 the info and hpe 2 cu l8ter' isn't going to make the admissions tutor look forward to the meeting and the tutor really DOESN'T LIKE BEING SHOUTED AT!!!!!!!!

- ✔ **Be concise and to the point.** The tutor doesn't want to know why your health promotion project on smoking has helped you understand addictive tendencies in teenagers, he wants to know why you've sent the email. Keep your email to a few short paragraphs, each making a salient point.

✔ **Think about structure and layout.** Reading from a screen is more difficult than paper. Use short paragraphs and add a line space between each of them. Use numbers if you have several points for consideration.

✔ **Read before sending:** It's all too easy to click 'send' immediately after writing the email without double-checking for errors. Re-reading your email helps you catch any mistakes and see the email through the eyes of the admissions tutor. You may wish to alter the emphasis or change a word to avoid any misunderstanding.

You can designate an email address on your UCAS application form. This address will be used by universities to communicate with you. Regular checks to your email account keeps you updated on the progress of your application.

Telephone manner

Nursing involves using the telephone as a way of communicating important information, and is often the only mode of communication used with some clients and families. Although you are taught on the programme how to develop your telephone manner, admissions tutors expect you to already have some basic skills.

The admissions team forms an impression of you based on your conversation. Just because you talk to them outside of the interview situation doesn't mean they don't use the opportunity to assess your suitability. They may write notes of the conversation in your file; make sure these are positive notes!

Here are some telephone tips:

✔ Always introduce yourself properly at the beginning of the conversation; likewise always ask for the person by name if they haven't introduced themselves. This way you both know who's speaking with whom.

✔ Speak clearly and in your natural voice. Take your time, pace your words and talk in a precise manner.

✔ Stick to the point. You can write down what you want to say in advance.

✔ Don't use slang or colloquialisms, because these can be misinterpreted, and certainly don't raise your voice, swear or become argumentative.

✔ Allow the listener to respond to your questions and don't talk over them. You can repeat what they've said if you haven't understood them the first time.

✔ Have a pen and paper at hand so you can jot down any advice or information.

✔ End the call in a courteous and polite manner even if you aren't happy with how the conversation has gone.

✔ If you're leaving a message, follow the rules in the preceding bullets. Leave a short message and remember to give your contact number. Clarity is important here, because a rushed telephone number is often hard to understand. Avoid phoning from a mobile phone in a busy environment.

Body language

On many occasions during the progress of your application you may meet with university staff. These are valuable opportunities for the admissions team to assess whether you have the beginnings of a student nurse.

Body language is a form of non-verbal communication, and the admissions tutor can read much from what you're saying through your actions and bodily responses. Focus on these two key areas:

✔ **Posture:** This speaks volumes about how you're feeling, giving a general indication of interest, confidence and mood. To create a happy, relaxed image, sit in a relaxed pose, with your head tilted slightly and your legs set apart. Ignore any distractions (especially your mobile – turn if off!) and focus on the other person or people with whom you're talking.

✔ **Personal space:** How close you stand to somebody is very important in making the right impression. You probably subconsciously make a decision as to the closeness; for example, with someone you care for you may stand close enough to embrace or touch them, whereas with someone unfamiliar you stand farther away.

Physical closeness says much about your relationship with others and also your sensitivity to other people's feelings. Standing closer may indicate a range of emotions from friendliness and confidence to aggressive posturing or poor social awareness. Stepping further away could indicate your wish to disengage from the person or that you are anxious and hesitant. You don't want to appear over-familiar, but at the same time you don't want to give the impression of not being interested either. A neutral position approximately a metre from the person offers the best solution.

Chapter 6

Gaining Care Experience

- -

In This Chapter

▶ Finding out what experiences could be useful to your application

▶ Exploring the range of experiences available

▶ Discovering what personal experience has to offer

- -

*I*f you're like most applicants, your decision to become a nurse is based on some meaningful encounter you've had with the health service. Very few candidates suggest their desire to be a nurse stems from dressing up in a nurse's outfit as a child . . . but admissions tutors still find a few! It is more probable that you've been a patient yourself, have had a family member need nursing or you already work within the care sector.

Although these initial encounters with nursing are positive – they've turned you onto a meaningful profession – a greater depth of interaction and experience within healthcare helps you understand the education and career choices you're making and demonstrate to admissions tutors that first-hand experience has taught you something about why you'd make a good nurse.

This chapter explains what care experience is and how it can improve your chances of success in your nursing school application. I show you the different types of care experience available and the potential advantages and disadvantages of each route. And finally, I explain the relationship of personal experiences to the wider nursing context, and the pitfalls of misunderstanding what's expected from candidates who use personal experience to support their application.

Understanding the Role of Care Experience

Whether universities require care experience and expect references, welcome it, or say only that such experience is desirable, in essence care experience improves your chances of getting a place on a nursing course.

But care experiences are only a means to an end, and not the end itself.

Most candidates undertake care experience in order to make their application forms look impressive. And that's fine as far as it goes, but simply showing up and ticking a box doesn't necessarily make you a winning candidate in the eyes of admissions tutors.

 The admissions tutor's view of the role of experience in the admissions process is different from that of many candidates. We see experience as a way for students to gain knowledge and understanding of caring and how nursing fits into the wider context of healthcare. Tutors don't view candidates' experiences as isolated events, but as a window to understanding what nursing is, how the profession works and the various roles and characteristics of nursing. In effect, admission tutors see experience as a starting point to develop further understanding, and they explore the meaning that each applicant has gained from her experiences.

When reviewing care experience, an admissions tutor asks of each candidate:

- ✔ Has she recognised what personal gains she has achieved?

- ✔ Does she understand how this experience supports a wider understanding of nursing?

- ✔ Has the experience permitted her to identify the positive attributes of a nurse, and is she able to recognise these attributes in herself?

- ✔ Through this experience, how did the applicant demonstrate what she has to offer nursing?

 View experience as a way to gain a personal insight into nursing and self-awareness of how nursing may affect you. Use your experiences as a trial run before the real thing and to understand whether nursing meets your expectations.

Putting a Plan Together

With so many opportunities available, gaining the most appropriate learning experience can be something of a challenge. You need to focus on what you want to gain from the experience and how the experience will support your application to nursing.

Providing a one-size-fits-all recommendation on the amount and type of experience each university wants to see is difficult. Every applicant has a different starting point, and the best advice is tailored to your personal requirements. So book yourself onto a university open day (see Chapter 9) and have a chat with the admissions tutor.

Applying for work experience requires plenty of advance planning. Many opportunities involve completing application forms and attending interviews. In certain organisations you may have to pass a health assessment or complete a Criminal Records Bureau check. And in some cases you join a waiting list! All these steps can seem like an ordeal in themselves, and they also take time – and sometimes cost money.

What you don't want to do is use all your resources securing work experience only to find it doesn't meet your expectations or help you secure that university offer. Ideally, you don't want to work for two weeks with a charity for learning disabilities if you want to become an adult nurse, and likewise it may not be the best experience to work in a care home for people with dementia if you're applying to be a student of child nursing.

Before starting your hunt for work experience, find out exactly what your chosen universities require. For example, one university may be quite happy for you to work a few hours a week in a local charity shop, but another university may expect you to demonstrate more patient contact.

When you know the university's requirements, work out what experience best fits your needs by asking yourself these questions:

- ✔ Which field of nursing are you interested in?

- ✔ What experiences do you already have that are useful to this field? What types of experience do you need to fill the gaps?

- ✔ If you're attending a school or college course, does this have provision for work experience?

- ✔ Can you afford unpaid experience or do you need an income?

- ✔ Do you want this experience to last several months or just a few weeks?

- ✔ How many hours a week can you dedicate to the experience?

- ✔ Are you able to work unsociable hours, or are there restrictions to when you can undertake the work experience?

The answers to these simple questions help you plan your experience, and they help organisations understand your requirements. For instance, being flexible with your time may mean that an organisation can offer a few hours a week over a longer period of time rather than a single two-week block.

You normally apply to university approximately ten months before the start of the course (check out Chapter 1 for a complete timeline). Being able to write on your application form that you have care experience means planning ahead. You may need to have gained experience a good one to two years before completing the application form.

Working within the NHS

The National Health Service (NHS) is the most well known of all healthcare providers in the UK and is probably the organisation that you've imagined yourself working within. The NHS is so ingrained into UK health culture that unless you've experienced healthcare in other countries, you couldn't imagine life without it. We may all grumble about waiting times for hospital appointments or the difficulty it takes to see a dentist, but few would dispute that when in urgent need, the NHS means access to medical or nursing care that can be both immediate and efficient.

The NHS is the world's largest publicly funded provider of healthcare, and in the UK it's the biggest single employer. Consisting of over 300 organisations, the NHS covers every spectrum of healthcare, from antenatal screening to end-of-life care, and employs healthcare professionals from every specialty (nearly 50 per cent of its workforce are clinically qualified). What this means for you is that ample opportunity exists to experience care in a wide variety of clinical situations and to work alongside many healthcare professionals, not just doctors and nurses.

Weighing up the pros and cons

The NHS offers many opportunities to experience care in a wide range of different clinical settings. It's a big organisation, and this creates benefits and limitations.

Experience you can gain

By far the main benefit of gaining work experience in the NHS is having access to the healthcare system in its entirety. Not only does the NHS cover the whole lifespan, but it also offers a service for every conceivable ailment, illness or condition. You can observe an infant being assessed by a health visitor through to a centenarian having her eyesight checked by an optometrist. Likewise, you can be part of the healthcare team in the patient's own home, a community health centre or in acute hospital settings. Essentially, the opportunities are endless: so long as you plan well, you should gain your desired experience.

Looking beyond the physical environment in which you work and those individuals that you meet, the experience offers a great introduction to the diversity of the organisation and how it ticks. You can gain valuable understanding that caring isn't just about doctors and nursing, but relies on effective working relationships between other healthcare professionals and the myriad of other jobs and careers.

Student nurses spend the majority of their education working within the NHS. Gaining NHS work experience brings you into contact with these students, and they can be a wealth of information on the do's and don'ts when applying for nursing . . . far better than reading any book or talking to admissions tutors.

Limitations

That the NHS is such a diverse organisation can have its drawbacks. Often departments can appear to work in isolation from others, and very much concentrate upon their own specialism. Should you gain experience in one particular area, this can give you a good insight on nursing for those specific patients, but may not give a full overview of the broad spectrum of nursing.

Finding work can also be a slog. Identifying where to go and who to contact in order to get the right advice can be daunting. Despite all your best efforts, you might feel that you come up against a brick wall in your search for the right experience. Perseverance is the key to success, and you must expect to be passed from one person to the next or have a long wait for people to reply to your requests. Polite and gentle reminders usually work well.

Getting your foot in the door

The NHS recognises that the future of healthcare relies upon attracting the best-suited individuals, and so it uses work experience as a way to increase awareness of the career opportunities available. The organisation is very encouraging in helping arrange work experience; however, the level of support and the manner in which this help is organised differs between departments. Using your plan, you need to decide which approach is best when making your request for work experience.

Work experience while in school or college

The NHS works closely with colleges and schools to allow students to gain work experience in healthcare. Many of the health science courses require students to undertake a set amount of work-based learning and you attend clinical environments as planned by your course tutor. Students often need to complete work place assignments and portfolios, and these usually go towards the award of your qualification. These health-related courses are directed mainly at 16- to 19-year-olds, and the length of the work experience can be quite minimal at only one to two weeks long.

This work experience is often observational only, which means you're limited to the amount of 'hands-on' care you get involved with. Sometimes it's difficult to choose which areas of clinical practice you can go to, so you may end up working in a nursing home and not accident and emergency! If you're planning to undertake some study before applying to university, check out which courses have healthcare experience built into them.

The NHS has a dedicated website for students that contains *The Smart Guide to Finding Work Experience in the NHS,* at www. stepintothenhs.nhs.uk.

Voluntary work

You can volunteer for the NHS to gain unpaid experiences of healthcare. Most organisations within the NHS have a procedure for supporting volunteers and find them a valuable asset to assisting professional staff in clinical environments.

Volunteers are actively involved with patients, and often assist with reminiscent sessions, playing games, talking, helping with drinks and sometimes feeding. You aren't expected to undertake personal care, such as washing and toileting, and nor are you involved in nursing care. The amount of time spent volunteering is quite flexible and could be between a few hours to a couple of days a week.

If you have experience of specific conditions or illnesses, you may find that these help you gain voluntary experience and that you're more involved with patients.

The NHS Choices website offers further advice for those considering volunteering, at www.nhs.uk/Livewell/volunteering/Pages/Howtovolunteer.aspx.

Paid work

Gaining paid work experience requires an extra level of planning. You need to research the local NHS organisations for job vacancies and develop your CV to its best potential.

Getting a job as a healthcare assistant

The most popular choice for gaining paid work is to become a *healthcare assistant*. Healthcare assistants work under the guidance of healthcare professionals, in this case nurses. You don't need any prior nursing experience because training is offered; however, you're expected to have a minimum level of education such as GCSEs. Roles vary slightly between employers, but because they involve attending to the personal care of patients, you need to be 18 years or older to apply. Personal care includes:

✔ Assisting with toileting

✔ Bed making

✔ Feeding and giving drinks

✔ General comfort

✔ Helping with walking and moving

✔ Washing and dressing

Extended roles for experienced healthcare assistants after training these could include nursing care such as:

✔ Administration of medicines (under supervision of qualified staff)

✔ Advanced feeding procedures

✔ Monitoring clinical conditions, such as blood pressure, pulse, respirations and temperature

✔ Simple wound dressing

Look for healthcare assistant posts because these give you good experience opportunities (see the nearby sidebar 'Getting a job as a healthcare assistant'). The posts generally have a higher level of clinical activity than the other types of NHS experience, and healthcare assistants undertake personal and nursing care. Many roles also include additional training in nursing procedures, such as monitoring blood glucose.

You have two main ways of gaining paid work:

✔ **Apply to an advertised post for a specific clinical area such as a medical ward or a community team.** Having a specific area to work means that you get to know the patients and staff and you have a set number of hours to work as part of your contract.

✔ **Apply to the nurse bank.** A *nurse bank* is a team of nurses and healthcare assistants whose role is to support the permanent nursing team when gaps appear in the workforce due to sickness, annual leave or busy times. Flexibility is the key here, because you can choose the days and hours that you can work. On the nurse bank you can expect to move around different clinical areas and you don't necessarily work in the same area or with the same team all the time.

The NHS has a website to advertise their job vacancies at www. jobs.nhs.uk. Local hospitals also have their own websites on which they advertise vacancies.

Turning to the Private Sector

The NHS is by far the largest provider of healthcare, but it's by no means the only provider. Independent organisations have an important role to play and are an accepted part of today's health-care system. The historical perception of the private sector is of a health system for the wealthy or for those people who need to be cared for in nursing or residential homes. These views are largely outdated, and although elements of these roles remain true, today you find the NHS and independent organisations working alongside each other to deliver care to the same group of patients and clients.

Weighing up the pros and cons

You can gain a wealth of experiences outside the NHS that helps towards a successful application. A wide variety of experience is available in the independent healthcare sector, and some of it is going to be more relevant to nursing than others, so you need to carefully select your experiences.

Have a browse of these websites to get a feel for the opportunities available:

- ✓ **Volunteering England:** www.volunteering.org.uk/
- ✓ **Scotland's centre for volunteering:** www.vds.org.uk/
- ✓ **Volunteering in Northern Ireland:** www.volunteering-ni. org/
- ✓ **Wales Council for Voluntary Action:** www.wcva.org.uk/
- ✓ **Volunteering in hospices:** www.helpthehospices.org.uk/ getinvolved/volunteering/

Experience you can gain

All private healthcare organisations work for and with the public, so you can gain valuable experience of working with patients, clients and their carers. The manner in which the care is delivered varies quite considerably. This gives you valuable experience of working with vulnerable or ill patients and helps you understand their feeling towards health and nursing. It also helps you to assess your people skills.

Choosing your experience wisely gives you the opportunity to work alongside qualified nurses and give hands-on care. This gives you real-time experience of some of the roles that student nurses are expected to perform plus insight into how care is delivered in the independent sector. This is useful information to have to help develop your application.

Student nurses are given the opportunity to work in the independent sector. Using your experiences within this sector can help prepare your application. Showing an appreciation that nursing doesn't just happen in the NHS demonstrates to admissions tutors that you have a broad understanding of our healthcare system in the UK.

Limitations

Some areas of the private sector, such as residential nursing homes, don't offer the same level of nursing care as hospitals. If you gain experience in a setting without a good degree of nursing then you may find it more difficult in your application to explain what you feel the nurse's role is or what will be expected of students.

Getting your foot in the door

You need to focus on roles that give you insight into caring or the nursing profession. Becoming a healthcare assistant (see the earlier sidebar 'Getting a job as a healthcare assistant') allows you to experience the hands-on care of a patient in one of three areas: independent hospitals, independent nursing and residential care, and agency nursing.

If you're studying a healthcare course at school or college you may have some scope to gain experience in a care setting as part of your course. Chapter 3 explains this in more detail.

Independent hospital experience

Depending upon the size of the organisation, independent hospitals can offer similar nursing experiences to the NHS. Some of the larger organisations have an extensive portfolio of care, which often focuses on acute surgical services. Many of these organisations care for NHS patients to reduce waiting lists or if specific investigative procedures are required, and so you can gain useful insight to the collaborative nature of healthcare.

In private hospitals you can experience close contact with patients and undertake both personal and nursing care. You experience nurses working in a variety of settings and gain insight to their many roles and responsibilities.

Independent nursing and residential care experience

This sector includes a range of organisations, from the very large UK-wide ones through to smaller companies with only a few homes, and then the single privately run homes.

You need to know the difference between a nursing and a residential home:

- **Nursing homes** provide hands-on nursing care and require qualified nurses to be continuously available to the patients. Here your experience can include clinical interventions such as specialised feeding and wound dressing. Working as a healthcare assistant, you'd be expected to deliver personal care but would also gain insight into the nurse's role in support of the patient.

- **Residential homes** base care upon a social model, and the residents don't necessarily require nursing intervention. These homes work towards maintaining the normality of home life and concentrate on the usual activities that people take for granted, such as entertainment and socialising. As a healthcare assistant, you can expect to participate in such activities and give personal care. Usually, you have only a limited exposure to nursing care.

Quite often homes are multi-purpose and provide both nursing and residential care. Both types of home have a close working relationship with community services, and you can gain an understanding of what care is available in the community and how nurses fit into the community team.

Unless you know where you want to work, searching for vacancies with each individual organisation can be quite laborious. To start your search, use a dedicated search engine such as Carehome – www.carehome.co.uk/care_search.cfm.

Newspapers are also a good source of information for vacancies in the smaller homes in your local area.

Working for private agencies

Private nursing agencies aim to offer suitably qualified nurses and care assistants to healthcare providers to cover any temporary gaps in their workforce. They work on the same principle as the

NHS nurse bank (see the earlier section 'Working within the NHS') but on a broader scale. The agencies don't have a permanent place of work, and employees travel to where they're needed. Many agencies offer help in hospitals, nursing and residential homes and places such as schools, mental health units and prisons. Your role would be to support the qualified nurse, which often entails a mixture of personal and nursing care.

The advantage of agency work is that you have flexibility in choosing when you work and for how long. Many care workers gain experience in a wide range of clinical environments, which can often include NHS hospitals, private nursing homes and patients' own residences. On the downside, working for a nursing agency can be quite an experience in itself, and you need to be a robust character to work in unfamiliar environments with different staff and unknown patients.

Volunteering for a Charity

Charities are voluntary organisations that offer a service to the public. They are usually started by a group of people who have a similar interest in a particular issue, subject or concern. After a charity achieves a certain level of income, it's required by law to register with the Charity Commission. Approximately 180,000 charities are registered in England and Wales, with a similar number of unregistered charities.

Clearly, not all these charities are related to healthcare. However, thousands of charities do concentrate their resources on healthcare issues, offering plenty of scope for gaining care experience.

Weighing up the pros and cons

Volunteering for a charity is a great way of developing your social skills because you'll undoubtedly work with people and in teams. With so many charities to choose from, knowing which one best suits your needs can be difficult. Try to ensure you gain experience that has a caring element to it. On a positive note, working for charities generally gives you a lot of insight into people's lives, how they function within society, and how society views health issues.

Experience you can gain

Although you can gain physical care experience when working with charities, such experiences are rare. The care experience is more often on a social basis, giving you a very good understanding of how people cope with their condition or disease.

Charities are often set up to offer support and advice that people can't easily gain elsewhere, such as charities that support children with cancer and their families and charities offering shelters for the homeless. Choosing an appropriate charity and getting the right role can give you real insight into the quality of people's lives and help you appreciate how social wellbeing and health are connected. This experience widens your understanding of health and can help support your people skills and demonstration of what caring is.

Limitations

Some charities can be far removed from nursing and healthcare, and you may find it difficult to relate your experiences with nursing or the role of the student nurse. You probably won't have any physical contact with patients, and you could find that your role is supporting families and visitors. This may not achieve your goals for gaining healthcare-related experience.

Getting your foot in the door

Most people relate to charities in terms of fundraising. You often see groups of people undertaking bizarre and exceptional activities to get you to relinquish your money. Although these are very honourable actions, they offer little valuable experience when supporting your application to nursing, so don't think running the marathon dressed as a canary contributes care experience to your application!

Charities rely upon volunteers to assist with the everyday running of their business, and this is where you can get good experience. Roles vary according to the nature of the charity, so think carefully about what experiences you're hoping to gain and which charities can provide them (the earlier section 'Putting a Plan Together' helps you work out what you're looking for). For example, if you feel you would enjoy nursing the older person, then Age UK may be a good charity to work for. However, if your interest lies in learning disabilities, then Mencap is a better option.

Here are a few ways to identify charities that may interest you:

✔ If you don't know which charity you want to volunteer for, CharityChoice (www.charitychoice.co.uk) is an excellent starting point for finding out your options.

✔ To find out more about charities that you have in mind and identify relevant opportunities, use their website and plug their name into a search engine for other perspectives.

✔ Some charities have shops that can be resources for finding out about vacancies in your local area.

Building Personal Experiences

You need to address your own personal experiences of care and whether they have a place in supporting your application. Personal experiences are an essential ingredient in how you view nursing and what you expect to do as a nurse . . . or in some cases, not to do!

Personal experiences are often a double-edged sword. Whereas you'd expect that using these experiences supports your application, doing so can have the opposite effect.

On a positive note, personal experience can be useful in that it can help demonstrate what you and nursing have in common. You may be able to recall an experience when you've either been ill yourself or have had family members need nursing care. Reflecting on the occasions you have thought 'I can do that' or 'that job seems very rewarding', you recognise some of the characteristics of the nurse in yourself. Nothing's wrong with being inspired by these experiences to pursue nursing.

But on a negative note, personal experiences mean that, as a consumer of care, you can be very subjective in your understanding of nursing. You may think nurses are great and that nursing is wonderful without any appreciation of the wider context of nursing. You push objectivity to one side and have little understanding of what the nursing profession is about.

If you want to use personal care experiences to support your application then you need to be aware that a subjective view can cloud your judgement of nursing, and it's possible that you may give an impression that you have unrealistic aspirations.

Rather than describing the personal care in detail, identify the aspects of the personal care that meant most to you in a professional manner. For example, perhaps the nursing staff treated you in a dignified, professional way, maintaining your personal right to be involved in important care decisions. You can say that this is the type of professional you aspire to be.

Part III
Preparing to Apply

Top Five Core Subjects on Nursing Programmes

- ✔ **Bioscience.** You learn about science, looking at the anatomy of the body and examining in detail all the different organs and systems.

- ✔ **Sociology.** You focus on the structure and dynamics of society and how and why people's lifestyles impact upon their wellbeing.

- ✔ **Psychology.** You study behaviour, and how people think, act and feel. You need to understand both positive and negative reactions to illness to tailor your nursing care to the patients' needs.

- ✔ **Law and ethics.** You learn the legal boundaries of what a nurse can and can't do and understand health ethics.

- ✔ **Nursing care.** You explore the meaning of nursing, the theories and models of nursing and understand the context in which you deliver care. You learn how to assess patients, plan and deliver care, and evaluate the effectiveness of care.

Go to www.dummies.com/extras/getintonursingschooluk for free online bonus content created especially for this book.

In this part . . .

✔ Know what to expect from your nursing programme – the theory and the practice.

✔ Get familiar with the teaching methods you'll experience.

✔ Meet the team who'll assess your nursing skills.

✔ Choose the best university for you, and make the most of open days.

✔ Find tips on getting the financial support you need at uni.

Chapter 7

Understanding the Nursing Programme

*E*ducating students to become future nurses is a complex process; it's not just a matter of attending lectures, passing exams and achieving your degree, but is about developing knowledge, assessing skills, meeting public expectations and following a political agenda. When designing a nursing programme there is a collaboration between the university that manage your studies and assesses your academic performance, the local healthcare providers that teach you clinical skills, and the Nursing and Midwifery Council (NMC), which determines how you should be educated and offers professional advice.

In this chapter, you see how these three organisations work together to produce a course of study that takes you from having no or minimal knowledge of care to, in three years, being a highly educated and clinically competent nurse. I explore the nature of the programme, how you're taught, how you learn, and how you're assessed, covering both the academic and clinical sides of the course. By the end of this chapter you have a good insight into the daily life of a student nurse.

Overviewing the Programme

You may hear of nurses who qualified from university with just a diploma or know a nurse who trained the 'traditional' way without any academic qualification. Many such nurses are out there, but you have only the one option – to study at degree level. From 2013 all nursing student have to undertake a degree programme to register as a nurse.

All nursing programmes teach you to degree level and prepare you for registration as a nurse. Look out for these terms that universities use when describing degrees:

- ✓ **BSc or BN degree:** The B means that it's a bachelor degree, the lower of the three degree levels (the others being master and doctor). The Sc means *science* and relates to the area of study. The N is for *nursing*.

- ✓ **Ordinary and honours degrees:** For the honours degree you undertake some additional study and assessment. Both degrees require you to study for three years and both make you eligible to register with the same nursing qualification. Given the choice, an honours degree looks a little better on your curriculum vitae (CV).

- ✓ **Pre-registration programme:** A programme for students who don't have a nursing qualification and aren't yet registered with the NMC.

- ✓ **Undergraduate programme:** A course leading to the achievement of a degree. You become a graduate when you pass the course.

Nursing courses are a minimum of three years in length and at the end you have two qualifications:

- ✓ **An academic award:** The university gives you an award, usually at a graduation ceremony, to say that you've achieved the level of bachelor degree.

- ✓ **Eligibility to register with the NMC**: You then have the option to register and work as a qualified nurse. This doesn't happen automatically, and you need to apply directly to the NMC. It is a straightforward procedure and the university helps you.

Nursing is a *vocational* programme of study, which means it involves both academic study and work experience. The split between theory and practice is even. You also have the option to include 300 hours of simulation learning that you complete either in a campus setting or in practice.

The following sections give you a broad overview of how universities structure and deliver the nursing course.

Understanding the NMC requirements

The NMC has a set of pre-registration standards that must be followed by universities. The standards describe in detail what students must achieve before they can register as a nurse. These requirements are built into the programme and include:

✔ **Time to complete the course:** For a full-time course the NMC expects you to complete in five years, which seems like a long time but can pass by very quickly. Unforeseeable circumstances are usually the cause of students not completing in time; for example, taking time out due to accidents or to care for a member of the family. Maternity leave is usually up to one year, but subsequent childcare can cause problems and prolong the course. Some students who find themselves pregnant twice on the programme struggle to meet the time limits.

✔ **Total hours of study:** The NMC requires that you complete 4,600 hours of study by the time you complete the programme. Many students think this is a university requirement and that lecturers are just being pedantic when adding up hours. It is, however, an important aspect of the programme and students encounter problems registering as a nurse when they haven't studied for enough hours, due to illness, for example. Students who haven't logged enough hours have to make up the hours either during the year or at the end of the course.

✔ **Nursing experience:** The NMC makes it clear that students must experience different types of nursing; otherwise you could complete the course and have cared for only one type of patient. In each field of nursing students are expected to experience caring for:

- Babies

- Children and young people

- Pregnant and postnatal women

- People with learning disabilities

- People with long-term problems

- People with mental health problems

Students are also required to experience a range of clinical environments, including care in the community and nursing in hospital settings. For adult nurses, the care of medical and surgical patients is also essential.

Students must experience care delivery through the 24-hour cycle and over the full 7-day period. Nursing isn't a 9–5, Monday-to-Friday job, and students' experiences must reflect the unsocial aspects of care delivery.

Surveying the academic teaching methods

During the course you study much of your theory hours on the university campus. Although each university has its own innovative ways of teaching, there are general ways in which you are taught:

- ✔ **Lectures:** Teacher-led sessions in which an expert in the subject provides information, often using visual aids. The teacher doesn't have to be a lecturer; the expert may be someone working in her speciality, such as a nurse from practice, a religious leader or a lawyer. Lectures are often used to give guiding principles on the topics under discussion and can be presented to a large number of students – 150 students in one lecture hall isn't uncommon. This does mean that interaction is quite limited.

- ✔ **Small-group work:** Students are divided into small teaching groups that can range between 15 and 30 students per group. These teaching groups often explore in depth the information given at lectures. Small-group work can be led by the teacher, but often the students themselves are involved in how the sessions are delivered. There is much more interaction between the teacher and the students, and opportunities exist to explore concepts and individual opinions.

- ✔ **Blended learning:** This approach to teaching and learning is about combining the traditional taught sessions with advanced e-learning methods. Students have contact with teachers but undertake much of their learning time using online resources. The resources can be a mixture of the universitiy's own e-learning packages and also external internet-based programmes. The advantage of blended learning is that students have flexibility as to when they complete work. They can work off campus and submit assessments electronically.

- ✔ **Reading time:** Most degrees have a considerable amount of reading time built into the timetable. For nursing students the reading time may not be so significant, but there will still be periods, either days or weeks, that are dedicated to self-directed study. The intention is for students to read around the subjects and build up a knowledgeable understanding of the concepts and issues. You can't learn all you need to know in the classroom, and students are expected to spend time reading books and articles.

- ✔ **Simulation:** Universities have their own *clinical skills suites* – teaching areas, normally on campus, that are designed to reflect a clinical environment such as a ward or the patients' own home. These suites contain the same equipment and materials found in clinical practice, and they place the student into a situation that mirrors clinical practice. Occasionally, actors, tutors or other students act as patients, although there are also mannequins that are very lifelike. Students can apply the knowledge they've gained in lectures to the clinical situation in a more safe and relaxed atmosphere than being out in a true clinical setting.

Universities place the responsibility for learning very much on you. Support is offered but you have to own your education. Reviewing your study skills now, by genning up on anatomy, physiology and numeracy, will help you once you get to university.

Considering patterns of work

The nursing programme is a combination of academic study on campus and clinical experience in practice. But how do these two work together and what does the combination mean for your daily routine?

Looking at modules

Learning is often delivered through a series of modules. Each module has a theme and all the teaching develops that theme in relation to nursing. The modules have academic credits attached to them that indicate how many hours of study and which assessments are needed to complete the module. At the end of the year the university adds up all the credits, and if you've passed enough credits, you progress to the next year.

Table 7-1 gives an example of modules for the first year.

Table 7-1	Example Modules for Year 1	
Title	**_Credits_**	**_Assessment_**
Module 1: Fundamentals of Nursing Care	10	Multiple choice questions
Module 2: Learning in the University and in Practice	10	Essay
Module 3: What Is Nursing?	10	Essay
Module 4: Developing Nursing Knowledge	20	Exam
Module 5: Introduction to Professional Practice	60	Skills

Notice that Module 5 has many more credits than the others; in fact, it has the equivalent number of credits as all the other four put together. That's because in this example the first four modules are theory modules and the fifth is the practice module – this meets the requirement that you spend 50 per cent of your time on theory and 50 per cent on practice. Here, Module 5 is a long module that runs right across the whole year, alongside the four other modules, and is the credit you get for all of your clinical experiences.

Mixing theory with practice

How you gain clinical experiences depends on your university and the local healthcare providers. Each university has its own way of managing your time in practice. Here are a few typical examples:

Example 1: Distinct periods

Week	1	2	3	4	5	6	7	8
	T	T	T	T	P	P	P	P

In this example the weeks are evenly distributed throughout the module between theory (T) and practice (P). Students have a period of teaching that covers relevant nursing concepts and then they attend clinical placement for an equal amount of weeks.

Example 2: Mixed periods

Week	1	2	3	4	5	6	7	8
	T	T	P	P	T	T	T	P

In this example over the eight-week period there's more theory than practice, but by the end of the programme the pattern would reverse, giving an equal ratio of hours overall.

Example 3: Integrated weeks

Day	Mon	Tues	Wed	Thurs	Fri	Sat	Sun
	P	T	T			P	P

This example demonstrates an approach where you work in practice and have taught sessions within the same week. It is a good way to help students relate theory to practice, and allows students to get regular support from tutors. Notice that the students work at the weekend here, with days off on a Thursday and Friday; this meets the NMC requirement of experiencing care delivery over a seven-day span.

Working out the hours

When you work full-time academic hours you work less than when working full-time in a job. The hours spent in the classroom vary, depending on the module content and the style of teaching, but they average anywhere between 10 and 25 hours per week studying on campus. Remember you're expected to be undertaking self-directed study during the week too . . . in other words, revision! So it's quite reasonable to be putting in a full 37.5 hours between teaching and revising each week.

When working in practice you're expected to work a variety of shift patterns that reflect the manner in which nurses deliver care. Because you're not a permanent member of the nursing team you have some flexibility in your hours and some choice over the days that you work. However, as part of developing your teamwork skills, you're expected to work similar shift patterns to the other nurses.

A typical working week is 37.5 hours and can include:

- ✔ **Monday to Friday, 9–5:** Normal working hours for students working in hospital day units, GP practices or alongside district nurses or health visitors in the community.

- ✔ **Early shift starting at 7 a.m. and finishing at 3 p.m.:** A typical morning shift in a hospital environment when nurses take over from the night staff.

- ✔ **Late shits from 1 p.m. to 9 p.m.:** The afternoon shift for a hospital ward. You care for the patients until the night staff take over.

- ✔ **The night shift from 8.45 p.m. to 7.15 a.m.:** You work a number of night shifts during your training, but not excessively or regularly.

- ✔ **The 12-hour shift from 8 a.m. to 8 p.m.:** This pattern of shift work has become quite popular because although you work a longer shift you get an extra day off each week. Some students find this shift very exhausting, both physically and mentally. Some universities argue that students are in placement for a learning experience, and that after 8 hours work, this is compromised.

As a student you don't have to work unsocial hours such as bank holidays, Christmas and Easter, but your clinical mentor will want you to be part of the team. Plan your commitments in advance and be flexible with your shifts and the nurses will be very accommodating.

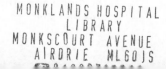

Focusing on Academic Study

On a nursing programme you can expect to study many health-related subjects, but unless you've studied health and social care, psychology or a science at school or college, do you know what you're likely to be learn about in the university classroom? Many universities don't expect you to have studied health-related subjects before applying for nursing, but the admissions team expect you to have some understanding of the course content.

Nursing follows a *social* model of learning, which means many subjects look at how people live, why lifestyles impact on health and how local and national policies impact on health and wellbeing. This is quite different to the *medical* model, which concentrates very much on the illness or the condition and its impact upon the body.

Seeing the breadth of subjects covered

Here are some examples of core subjects on nursing programmes:

- ✔ **Bioscience.** You learn about science, looking at the anatomy of the body and examining in detail all the different organs and systems. The anatomy and physiology of the body is discussed in-depth so you appreciate normal function. You're then introduced to the pathophysiology of the body, how abnormal function happens and what this means to the patient. This often includes discussing illness and conditions and their relationship to the different body parts.

- ✔ **Sociology.** Focuses on the structure and dynamics of society and how people experience life. Its usefulness to nursing is in explaining how and why people's lifestyles impact upon their wellbeing. Sociology is a very important aspect of nursing because you can't really care for your patient if you don't understand who they are, how they live and what their attitude towards health is.

- ✔ **Psychology.** Mainly the study of behaviour, psychology explores how people think, act and feel. It is the scientific study of the mind, and you study this subject to explore how ill people react to their illness. You need to understand both positive and negative reactions to tailor your nursing care to the patients' needs.

- ✔ **Law and ethics.** There are legal boundaries to what a nurse can and can't do, and for yourself and your patient, you must know and understand the legal implications of nursing. At the same time, understanding health ethics is vital to appreciating the moral and professional principles of caring for the vulnerable and sick.

✔ **Research.** Not a subject you may have expected as core teaching, but research and understanding sources of evidence go to the heart of nursing. You can only be a good nurse if you practise good-quality care, and to do this you must use the best available evidence. This subject helps you develop a critical thinking mind that constantly questions your practice and looks for ways to improve your care.

✔ **Nursing care.** Central to your development and uses all the preceding subjects and those not mentioned to inform and support your understanding of nursing care. This subject explains the meaning of nursing, explores theories and models of nursing and helps you understand the context in which you deliver care. You explore how to assess patients, plan and deliver care, and evaluate the effectiveness of care.

Taking academic assessments

For each module you go through an assessment, based on which credits are awarded. You're assessed using a range of methods that allow you to demonstrate your understanding and knowledge of the subjects taught:

✔ **Academic essay.** A popular method of assessment; you write an essay against a set of guidelines. In your essay you inform the reader that you understand the topic in question. Various types of essay exist, such as reflective accounts in which you review a nursing experience and critiques of nursing concepts.

✔ **Presentation.** Allows more creativity in the way you present your knowledge and understanding – a great way of explaining nursing care in your own words if you don't like essays or exams. You deliver presentations orally or as a poster presentation, and often as group.

✔ **Exam.** Every student loves an exam, right? So of course most universities throw a few in to keep you happy! Exams take an example of your performance to predict how well you're developing. The nature of the exam may vary. You may need to show your expertise in a particular area, such as numeracy skills, or you may have a choice of questions across a range of topics. Some exams may be scenario based, in which you have to explore nursing care.

✔ **Observed structured clinical examinations (OSCEs).** Methods of assessment that review your clinical skills. You prepare carefully and then you demonstrate a skill in the clinical suite while the assessor observes. Typical skills in your first year include hand washing, recording a temperature and taking blood pressure. You're not just assessed on the clinical skill but also on your communication skills and professionalism.

Getting to Grips with Clinical Study

To become a nurse you must undertake clinical practice in a variety of environments and with a range of different patients. But don't worry – you're not just parachuted into a clinical area and expected to observe the nurses and learn the ropes. Your clinical study is as structured as your academic study.

In practice you work alongside healthcare professionals and your nurse mentor, whose role it is to ensure you have the right learning opportunities (for more on the mentor's role, see the later section 'Understanding the Roles of Staff Members'). These opportunities include looking after patients and delivering hands-on care plus observing interventions and treatments, getting involved with patient evaluations and supporting families and carers.

Covering the Essential Skills Clusters

The NMC makes it a requirement that you are assessed on your clinical aptitude and they set out these requirements in their *Essential Skills Clusters*. These clusters are a set of guiding principles on the evidence you need to provide when in clinical practice to show you're developing into a competent practitioner.

There are five Essential Skills Clusters (see the bulleted list that follows) and each has a number of criteria that you must achieve before progressing to the next year. Each year you have to meet a new and more difficult set of criteria for each cluster. Your nurse mentor bases your learning around these criteria when caring for patients.

Here's an example of the criteria for your first year of study:

- ✔ Care, compassion and communication:
  - Can apply the principles of confidentiality.
  - Uses clear communication skills both orally and written.
  - Respects diversity and individual preference.
- ✔ Organisational aspects of care:
  - Responds appropriately when faced with an emergency or a sudden deterioration of a patient's condition.
  - Acts within legal frameworks and local policies.
  - Knows own limitations of role, knowledge and skill.

✔ Infection prevention and control:

- Demonstrates effective hand hygiene.

- Follows local policy regarding dress code.

- Maintains a high standard of personal hygiene.

✔ Nutrition and fluid management:

- Follows food hygiene procedures.

- Can report a risk of a patient missing meals.

✔ Medicines management:

- Is competent in basic medicines calculations relating to tablets, liquid medicines and injections.

Assessing you in practice

Each criteria from the Essential Skills Clusters (see the preceding section) will be incorporated into a clinical portfolio that you take with you each time you go into practice. Be careful not to lose this document as it's your only record of your clinical practice ability for the entire year. This portfolio is used by your mentor when she assesses you. Your mentor assesses you in a number of ways:

✔ **Practical observation:** Very much like the OSCEs on campus (see the earlier section 'Taking academic assessments'), but these observations are with real patients. You're expected to work alongside other nurses delivering care to patients and supporting their families where appropriate. Situations are explained to you and opportunities are made available for you to practise your nursing skills against the Essential Skills Clusters. While you do this your mentor observes you and asks you questions.

✔ **Presentations:** Similar to those performed on campus (see the earlier section 'Taking academic assessments'), but this time in the clinical setting. You may be expected to look after a patient or a group of patients, plan and deliver their care and then present your understanding of that care to your mentor. You have to show you know the pathology of the condition and the psychosocial issues for the patient, and explain in detail the relevant nursing care.

✔ **Behavioural appraisal:** Alongside all your clinical skills assessments your mentor assesses your professional behaviour: how you conduct yourself in practice, engage with other healthcare professionals and present yourself to your patients. You develop the essential attitudes and behaviours for nursing (which I discuss in Chapter 5) in practice and you're assessed on your compassion, sensitivity and caring qualities.

Understanding the Roles of Staff Members

Teaching on the nursing programme is delivered by a team of academic lecturers. All the lecturers have appropriate skills and knowledge that is useful for your development. This team is often made up of nurse lecturers who have nursing and teaching quali- fications and whose nursing career is now in education. However, the team also include subject specialists who are not necessarily nurses; for example, scientists, sociologists and solicitors.

The core team is permanent and works full-time, but the university also invites specialists to speak as honorary lecturers and many of your sessions are taught by practising professionals who work in their relative professional and teach part-time. Using a wide variety of teachers ensures you receive the most appropriate and up-to- date knowledge possible.

Apart from teaching the academic lecturers also have other roles.

The academic tutor

Academic tutors are members of the academic staff you may go to when you need advice regarding the academic content of the module or programme. Academic tutors may be actively involved with assessing your academic work and may be allocated to you as an academic supervisor for your work. Academic tutors are specialists in the subject area being taught and do not have to be nurses. Your academic tutor:

- ✔ Allocates a supervisor to you for each of the academic modules.
- ✔ Offers guidance on the assessment criteria of the module.
- ✔ Gives support and supervision to help you prepare your submission.
- ✔ Assesses and marks your submitted work, and gives feedback.

The personal tutor

The *personal tutor* is a member of the academic staff who provides you with support and guidance throughout your nursing studies. You're allocated a personal tutor at the beginning of your studies and that tutor often follows your progress through the entire three years of the programme.

On nursing programmes it is customary for personal tutors to be nurses in the field that you intend to enter. You'll find that these tutors have a wealth of experience in clinical practice. There's a varied mix of specialities among the tutors so that all aspects of nursing are covered. For example, tutors have backgrounds in the following nursing areas: medical, surgical, intensive care, community and infection control. Many tutors will have also been managers and senior nurses.

These tutors have an active registration with the NMC. Many tutors continue to work in clinical practice as well as lecturing. They're a good source of inside knowledge that's well worth tapping into.

Personal tutors focus on supporting you in a *pastoral* role, considering your health and wellbeing while on the programme rather than your academic development, although they do tend to look at both. Typically, the personal tutor:

- ✔ Helps you to settle into your programme and manage homesickness.

- ✔ Directs you to the appropriate support for financial management.

- ✔ Helps to develop strategies to manage family pressures.

- ✔ Offers regular meetings to keep in touch.

- ✔ Monitors your levels of absence and sickness.

- ✔ Works with you on practice-related issues.

- ✔ Addresses any issues relating to your overall progress on the course.

- ✔ Gives guidance should your good character be brought into disrepute!

The nurse mentor

A *mentor* is almost always a registered nurse who offers experienced professional advice and support to junior members of a team. Nursing programmes use the mentorship system to support student nurses when in clinical practice. Nurse mentors are experienced individuals who take an interest in the nurturing of future nurses. When you go into practice you're allocated a nurse mentor for the time you're working in that clinical area and so have several mentors during your training as you have several different clinical experiences. Nurse mentors have two roles: as assessor and role model.

Clinical assessor

Your nurse mentor acts as your assessor for that clinical placement. They meet with you at the beginning of the placement and on a frequent basis throughout your stay to discuss your learning needs, plan your care experiences and monitor your progress. The nurse mentor:

- ✔ Plans your learning opportunities for the placement.

- ✔ Identifies any concerns or issues that you may have.

- ✔ Sets tasks and arranges experiences for you.

- ✔ Asks questions of you and assesseses your knowledge.

- ✔ Observes your caring and communication skills.

- ✔ Reviews your documentation and writes your progress reports.

Professional role model

Your mentor also acts as a role model for your professional development. Role modelling allows student nurses to observe experts undertaking their professional job. Role modelling is an effective teaching method in clinical practice, where there are increasing demands on the mentor's time. You get to:

- ✔ Develop a professional attitude through observing professionals.

- ✔ Learn from experienced and knowledgeable nurses.

- ✔ See theory applied to practice.

- ✔ Get closer to the nursing team.

Chapter 8

Exploring Universities

● ●

In This Chapter

▶ Thinking about the university's reputation

▶ Exploring the programme

▶ Considering location and accommodation

▶ Checking out the social side

▶ Using websites to help you research

● ●

*W*ith over 68 universities to choose from, finding the best match for your requirements may be a bit of a challenge. Universities differ in terms of course material, assessment methods, clinical practice experiences and the overall student experience. You need to take your time, undertake some research and plan a strategy to ensure that your decision is the best one for you. Choosing the right course at the right university requires some work, and this chapter offers assistance in pulling together your thoughts and ideas.

Although all universities offering nursing programmes follow the same Nursing and Midwifery Council standards for pre-registration education, no national curriculum exists and each delivers their programme in a different way. All universities promote themselves as student friendly and show you all the good reasons that you should choose them over others. Few universities give detailed information of the courses or the not-so-good points of studying there, so you have to do some detective work, reading between the lines and investigating the evidence to find out what being a nursing student at each university really means. In this chapter, I help you consider all the options, review the different opportunities and identify drawbacks.

Some students make the wrong decision and choose a university that doesn't suit them. Transferring between universities is a possibility, but no university can guarantee to find you a place. So focus on choosing the right university in the first instance, rather than holding on to the notion of transferring as a backup plan.

Probing Programme Particulars

Even though every nursing programme leads to registration as a nurse, you find that each university has its own way of running the course, assessing its students and managing the way you study. There are similarities across all universities as each course must meet the NMC rules and regulations; for example, every course requires students to spend time in clinical practice. But each university has a lot of scope to develop their own teaching, and this can have a big impact on your day-to-day learning.

When exploring universities, find out not only the structure of the course but also the finer details of how the course works, as it is often these details that have the biggest effect on your daily student activities.

Checking that the university offers the right course

Not all universities offer nursing courses, and those that do offer courses don't necessarily offer all the nursing fields. For example, far more places are available for adult nursing than for learning disabilities, which has very few places on offer. Obviously, universities can't run courses for just a few individuals, so you have less choice of university for the smaller fields. Table 8-1 outlines the number of universities offering courses in each field.

Table 8-1	Courses Available in Nursing Fields
Nursing Field	*Number of Universities Offering a Course*
Adult	Over 65
Mental health	Approximately 55
Child	Over 45
Learning disabilities	Approximately 33

Use UCAS course search to give you a quick calculation of how many universities teach your chosen nursing field.

Looking at length of study

The length of time is takes to study nursing depends upon your own circumstances and the course that you choose. All nursing programmes are offered as full-time courses, which means that you enroll as a full-time student and work the expected full-time academic hours. Previous enthusiasm to provide part-time or flexible routes in nursing has very much evaporated, except for in a few universities.

The following options are available:

- ✔ **Four-year programme:** A few universities offer a four-year programme leading to an honours degree. These longer courses are offered for different reasons. As a flexible route, the four-year programme means working fewer hours as a student over each year and this may suit you if you have to manage other commitments. Registering as a nurse takes longer, but you get to spread the same finances as a regular three-year programme over the four years.

  Some universities (Scottish mostly) offer a full-time four-year programme that gives you registration as a nurse after the third year and an optional fourth year to gain an additional specialist registration with the NMC. This is an ideal way to continue your academic studies and gain the specialist award before leaving university. But keep in mind that you need to be very focused on where you want your nursing career to lead in relation to the specialist award.

- ✔ **Three-year programme:** By far the most popular length of study for a nursing degree, and most three-year degrees offer the honours component. All fields of nursing offer this option to study, and you're classed as a full-time student. This option offers greater choice of university at which you can undertake your studies.

- ✔ **Two-year programme:** Offered by a few universities, this programme is an accelerated version of the three-year full-time programme. The option is designed for students with prior knowledge or experience and you need to have a good first degree in a healthcare-related subject. Alternatively, if you already have a nurse registration and wish to add another nursing field to your profile, then you can access this two-year programme. Sometimes this includes applicants who hold a registration in another country.

Requirements exist regarding the length of time you can study to become a nurse, and these alter slightly according to the programme details. The NMC requires all nursing students on a full-time programme to complete their studies within five years. Consider your long-term commitments before embarking on a full-time programme.

Noting start and finish dates

Give serious consideration to the actual dates of the course. Candidates who don't heed the dates that nursing programmes work to can seriously jeopardise their chances of success. In many instances nursing students don't work to usual university term dates.

For the 'normal' university student, the academic year is laid out in a straightforward manner and is easily to follow; the year essentially starts in September or October and concludes in May or June. The academic year is divided and subdivided as follows:

- ✔ **Semesters:** Each academic year is split into two *semesters*, a teaching period followed by assessments or examinations. Each semester is approximately 14 to 20 weeks in length. Semester 1 covers the period from September to December and Semester 2 from January to June.

- ✔ **Term times:** Terms are periods of study within the semesters that are separated by periods of no study (holiday time!). Typically, a year has three terms that give you holidays at Christmas, Easter and summer:

  - Michaelmas term: September to December

  - Lent term: January to March

  - Summer term: April to June

But for nursing students, the academic year isn't so straightforward, and how the programme fits into term times may vary. Nursing students have to meet university regulations on how much time they study, and so each module has a required amount of teaching time and self-directed learning hours. On top of this, the NMC requires students to complete a set number of hours before registering as a nurse. Achieving an academic qualification and a professional qualification means you have to work longer than other university students.

 When considering your university choices, check the following information:

- ✔ **When does the programme start?** It may start at the same time as all other students, but it could start two to three weeks earlier.

- ✔ **How often does the programme start?** Some universities have two intakes a year and this means you may start in September or October or alternatively in February or March. Your term time and annual leave is different depending on when you start the programme.

✔ **When are the annual leave dates?** Nursing students have leave over Christmas and Easter. However, other annual leave entitlements may not follow the academic pattern. Some nursing students work through the summer, and it is not unusual to be on campus or in placement during the June–August period. You may have leave when other university students are studying, and vice versa.

The academic year for a student nurse is much longer than for other university students. This is partly to do with the content and structure of the programme, but also to do with government requirements for eligibility of funding. Students are required to work a minimum of 42 weeks per year to receive the public funding for course fees and associated bursaries.

Universities develop their curriculum in advance. You can ask for approximate dates for starting the programme and leave entitlements throughout the first year. This information helps you make plans and manage commitments prior to commencing the programme.

Tallying study hours

Student nurses must undertake a minimum of 4,600 hours of study. This is a requirement of the NMC, and all universities have to ensure their students achieve this many hours before registration. The hours are split between academic study and clinical practice. The other NMC requirement is that nursing students have equal time between study and practice, and this 50/50 split is a recognised good feature of the programme.

The media fascination with nurse education being too academic is a myth. All universities place students in clinical practice for a minimum of 50 per cent of the entire programme. Overall, if you consider only the actual face-to-face contact hours between you and your lecturer and you and your clinical mentor, then clinical practice wins hands down. You spend more time with your mentor and the patients than you do with your lecturers.

With these excessive hours, your working week is much longer than that of other students. Some courses at university have only six hours of contact time with lecturers per week, with much of the study hours made up of reading time. It is usual for nursing students to have much more contact time, and you can expect to be in the classroom 15 hours per week. The hours you study and number of days each week that you're in the classroom alters according to the module and the curriculum design.

I only mention academic study hours in this section. Don't forget that when in clinical practice your working hours could be as much as 37.5 hours per week. Chapter 8 gives more details on patterns of work.

When exploring universities, find out how the taught part of the programme is managed. The admissions tutor can give you a sample timetable that shows the hours of study in the classroom. The following questions can help you think about the hours you work:

- ✔ Are you in the classroom every day of the week, or are there set days of study?

- ✔ How long is a typical teaching day in the classroom?

- ✔ How much 'self-directed study' is included each week (when you can work on your own, often off campus)?

- ✔ Are there set times for 'universitiy activities' such as sport?

Working in clinical practice

Half of your programme is working in clinical practice, so you need to know just how the university organises this and what it expects from you. When assessing courses, look at the following aspects:

- ✔ **Organisation of practice time:** Some universities place you in practice for many consecutive weeks, but others use shorter and more frequent clinical periods.

- ✔ **Patterns of work:** Do you have to work set weekends, a number of night shifts or evening shifts? Some flexibility exists for students at different universities, and knowing beforehand the level of unsocial hours you have to work helps you plan how to manage the commitment alongside other aspects of your life.

- ✔ **Where will you work?** The NHS is an obvious starting point, and you'll have to work in hospitals and in the community, but do any special or interesting clinical areas call out to you? Some universities link with regional specialist areas such as burns or cardiac units.

- ✔ **How far are you expected to travel and what arrangements are made if you use public transport?** Don't expect patients to be wheeled into the classroom; you need to visit them in their homes, at hospital and in community centres. At some universities visiting patients entails a trip of a few miles, but for others you could be facing an hour-long journey by bus.

Checking out the day-to-day structure

The programme has a real impact on your student experiences. Many students find university life to be quite demanding against their other commitments, and the day-to-day running of the course impacts on how you manage to balance family and social commitments with those of studying. Looking through prospectuses and reading through university websites give little indication of how the curriculum is structured on a daily level.

Plan your calendar so you can attend a few open days. All good universities have student ambassadors available for you to chat with. They're a great source of information when it comes to knowing the 'nitty gritty' aspects of daily life as a student nurse. (For more on open days, head to Chapter 9.)

Also ask the university for an example of the timetable. This gives you an idea of what your typical week will be like and helps your teaching. But do keep in mind that many universities have large healthcare departments that teach more than just nursing students. Teaching paramedics, midwives, physiologists and medical students causes some organisational difficulties when planning the use of clinical skill suites and going out into clinical practice. Be prepared to see creative timetabling!

Looking at Location

An important aspect in your choice is where the university is in the UK. Look on each university website and you'll see wonderful pictures of idyllic scenery or frenetic night-life, all suggesting that the university is a great place to be. But don't just take what you read at face value – think carefully about whether the location – where the university is in the country, its proximity to your home and the type of place it is – meets your needs and desires.

Being close to home, or far away?

Do you want to spread your wings and see life in another part of the country? Are you self-reliant and happy to support yourself and live an independent life away from family and friends?

Or are you a homebody? Do you need to be close to home to look after others? Many students have children and find moving across the country difficult to manage. Equally restrictive is the rise in students who are carers for elder members of the family.

Given the opportunity, studying away from home has advantages. You build independence and self-reliance; skills that you transfer into your professional work. Depending on where you're from, you may also find better job prospects exist away from home.

Finding the type of campus to suit you

Universities vary in size from the large metropolitan institutions with over 30,000 students to the smaller universities with only a few thousand students. Which do you prefer? Consider the following:

- ✔ The larger the university, the busier the environment. A good-sized campus provides lots of extra activities and there will be plenty of opportunities to mix with non-nursing students and get involved with student life.

- ✔ Some universities are split up into colleges and departments and based on separate sites. You may find that you have to travel between sites to access all the university services such as financial advice or essay support. Smaller universities may only have one campus with all facilities on the same site.

- ✔ The size of the university can impact on teaching styles. For example, some deliver many healthcare programmes and so you could find yourself undertaking shared learning in lectures of 150 or more students from all different healthcare programmes such as paramedics and physiologists.

Also think about:

- ✔ **Urban or green?** Do you like the night-life and is it important for you to enjoy your free time? Would a city-based university be your ideal location, or are you happy to have a more sedate pace to your student life? Would a smaller, more personal, campus suit you better?

- ✔ **Cost of living:** Some locations are more expensive than others. It may be a great idea to study in the bright city lights, but will your bursary keep up with your aspirations?

- ✔ **Access to fun stuff:** Are you a keen canoeist, a determined surfer or a theatre lover? Check the scope in the location to pursue your interests.

Getting there and back again

Consider the ease of travel back and forth to university:

✔ **By car:** Some universities have restrictions on car parking and don't allow students to park on the campus site. There may be designated parking off-campus and within walking distance. If parking is available, how much does it cost? Most universities apply parking charges that can add up to a hefty sum. Check whether car-sharing schemes are available for which you get a discount on parking charges.

✔ **By public transport:** Larger universities often have good train links and dedicated bus routes that make it easy to travel back and forth from your accommodation. Smaller universities may require you to be more organised if using public transport, or expect you to have your own transport.

✔ **By bike.** Many universities encourage cycling in and around campus and have schemes and facilities to encourage more cycling. They may work in partnership with local communities or authorities to provide cycle tracks and secure parking that may make your travelling less costly.

All universities work within the Equality Act and offer support to disabled students. This support may be more limited in some universities than others. Contact the disability team to find out availability of parking spaces and access to buildings.

Considering Bed and Board

The type of accommodation on offer can be a deciding factor in your choice of university. Most offer a good selection, but others may limit you to private landlords. Here are some considerations when looking at accommodation:

✔ **Do special arrangements exist for nursing students?** Some universities dedicate separate houses to healthcare students because of their unsocial shift work and long academic year.

✔ **How many years is the accommodation for?** Usually, university accommodation is only available for the first year and you have to find your own private accommodation in years two and three. What support will the university offer in helping you find alternative accommodation?

✔ **How many weeks is the accommodation for?** Student nurses work a longer academic year. You don't want to be thrown out of your house before your year ends.

✔ **What's the cost of accommodation?** All universities charge you to use their accommodation, but charges vary depending on the location of the university and the type of accommodation on offer. Having shared facilities, such as a kitchen and bathroom, is usually cheaper than having your own en suite facilities. Catered halls accommodation may not be cost effective if breakfast is served from 8 a.m. and you're expected to be in clinical practice at 7.

Each university has its own way of allocating accommodation. Check out websites early to find out how to apply.

Some students go for the halfway option and get the best of both worlds. Moving to a university within easy travel distance from the family home but far enough to be independent is a good way of settling into life on your own. You have the option of moving back home after the first year if private accommodation doesn't suit you, but bear in mind that clinical practice often starts early or finishes late, making a long journey home impractical.

Exploring Extra-Curricular Activities

Being a nursing student doesn't have to be all work and no play, and sometimes you take time out from studying to enjoy being a student. Many universities invest heavily in the social aspect of student life and encourage you to engage with non-study activities. Participation in extra-curricular activities is encouraged as a personal development opportunity. You build transferrable skills that are useful in employment, such as teamwork and communication, organisational and time-management skills. When choosing your university, the social side of things, and overseas training may be important to you.

Scoping social activities

Being involved with the social side of university life is entirely optional, but most students who do actively engage find that they're better prepared when it comes to applying for their first qualified nurse job. The social aspect of university life may not be high on your list of priorities when choosing a university, but it can give a clue as to how the university likes to work with students. Universities work hard to ensure their students have the right skills to improve your chance of employment and encourage you to get involved with university activities such as working with the student union, or in university shops, or being a student representative on committees.

Each university has a selection of sports and hobby clubs and probably a fitness and health centre too. Check out the website for a list of clubs available. You may be surprised at the variety!

Alternatively, the student union brings you into contact with the organisation of the university. If you want to develop your relationship with management and the running of the university then you'll find opportunities for getting involved with committees, becoming a student rep or working as student ambassadors so you can and have your say in the day-to-day practices of the nursing programme.

Overseas opportunities

Overseas placements make up part of some nursing programmes. They're a great way of seeing the world and developing your nursing knowledge and skills. When you study abroad you benefit from deeper engagement with different healthcare cultures and your understanding of the UK healthcare system is enhanced by your appreciate of global healthcare.

The Erasmus exchange programme supports student mobility throughout Europe. You get the opportunity to spend between 3 and 12 months in a European country experiencing the nursing care and health system for yourself. Financial aid is available, although you need to use some of your own money too, and you receive academic support while you're away. Check whether universities you're interested in are members of the scheme, and if so which European countries they are partner to.

Perusing Student Information Websites

When searching for your ideal university, a good point of call is to visit websites with relevant information for students. The information you find in a survey, for example, can be very useful in understanding what other people have thought about your chosen university and can remove some of the subjectivity that's crept into your ideas and thoughts.

Be sure to check out the following sources of information.

The National Student Survey (NSS)

Students in their final year of study are encouraged to evaluate their university and give their opinion about what they liked and disliked about their course. Conducted between February and April each year, over 200,000 students have participated in the survey since 2005 and commented on many issues that are important for you as you decide which university is best for you. The good news is that students rate nursing courses highly, and over 80 per cent of students have said they were happy with their student experience.

Here are some examples of statements that students are asked to rate their satisfaction against:

- I have been able to access general IT resources when I needed to.
- The library resources are good enough for my needs.
- Feedback on my work has helped me clarify things I did not understand.
- Staff have made the subject interesting.
- I have received sufficient help and support for my studies.

The results from the NSS are displayed on the Unistats website (http://unistats.direct.gov.uk), the official website for all the government statistics on universities.

Key information sets on Unistats

Universities submit key information in the same categories each year, which makes comparing universities like for like very easy. A useful feature of the website is the ability to select different universities for comparison so you can choose only those universities you're interested in and with a click of a button see how they compare.

Universities are required to give information on:

- The breakdown of the course between lectures, self-directed study and practice.
- The type of assessments on the course.
- Average salary six months after completing the course.
- The percentage of students in full-time employment six months after completing the course.

If you already know which university you are interested in but don't want to use the official website, visit the university website, which will advertise the Unistats on the relevant course pages.

Universities seek a good reputation, and league tables rank each accordingly to the statistics. These vary each year, and unless you're adamant that only the top university will do, the information in Unistats is generally sufficient to ensure your choice of university is of a good quality.

Discussion boards and forums

Chapter 11 gives much more detail about UCAS and how to use it to plan and submit your application. But the UCAS network YouGo (www.ucas.com/yougo) is also useful for finding out what people think of different universities and courses. There you find discussion boards and forums where you can get advice, listen to opinions and generally find out what others in the same position as you think.

If you're interested in students' opinions, also visit The Student Room (www.thestudentroom.co.uk). It's the largest student forum in the UK, covering students in sixth form and at college and university, so you can find likeminded people asking similar questions. Generalised help on topics include:

- ✔ Housing and accommodation.
- ✔ Keeping healthy.
- ✔ Study advice.
- ✔ Writing your personal statement.

Also look for forums specific to nursing and healthcare. At the last count there were over 32,000 messages on topics such as:

- ✔ Bursary for mature students.
- ✔ Good character statements and nursing.
- ✔ Nursing in London.
- ✔ Writing care experience in personal statements.

Considering the Competition

Nursing is a very popular profession. It is the most popular degree programme, with the number of applications to nurse degree courses (200,000 per year) exceeding those of all other university courses.

Part of the attraction is down to the generous financial support that nurses have historically enjoyed, with no academic fees and access to an NHS bursary. Another factor is the change in the academic level of education. Nurse education had originally been taught at diploma level, but over the last few years it's moved to all degree programmes.

Application numbers have increased year on year, and the rate of increase has been between 19 and 35 per cent depending on the UK country. The result is that gaining a student nurse place is a very competitive process, and many candidates will undoubtedly be disappointed.

However, with a bit of foresight, motivation and sheer willpower, you can be successful in your application. Understanding the competition and knowing how to play the game can give you the advantage over the other candidates. The following sections outline some strategies to consider.

Knowing what you're up against

Some fields of nursing are more popular than others, both in the number of places available and also the number of applications they attract. Table 8-2 offers an example of a university showing how many places are available for each field, the number of applications received and the ratio of applications to places.

Table 8-2   Ratio of Applications to Nursing Places

Field	Number of Places	Number of Applications	Ratio of Applications to Places
Adult	100	1,500	15:1
Child	12	300	25:1
Mental health	57	250	4:1
Learning disabilities	20	120	6:1

Your chances can improve quite considerably when you think about the application process. Candidates can make five choices on their application form, so the 200,000 applications to nursing school per year could be generated from just 40,000 candidates. These choices can be five separate universities for the same field, or a mixture of fields and universities. However, every candidates isn't successful with every choice. In addition, a successful candidate ultimately has to choose a first and second choice, thereby rejecting the other three options. These variables can improve your chance of success.

This means that lots of choices are made by fewer candidates, so although the initial ratio above appears very high, when taking into account that the candidate can only go to one university, the figures become less drastic. Candidates don't apply in such an easy and straightforward way: some only apply to a few universities and others apply for a mix of nursing fields at the same university, so the odds are never that simple. The important aspect here, though, is that it is highly likely that the applicant ratio represents a worst-case scenario and not your true opportunities.

Choosing a geographical area

Choosing a geographical area can improve your chances. Hospitals have different needs and develop their services accordingly, which means they need different numbers of nurses. Take a look Table 8-3 in which I show you the reduction in student places in different locations in the country.

Table 8-3	Reduction in Student Places in Different Locations
Location	*Reduction in Places*
Northern Ireland	19%
Scotland	12%
Wales	11%
England	9%
(North East	4%)
(West Midlands	19%)

The information helps you understand that the location of the university and the particular health needs of the population has an impact on student numbers. Considering your potential to move around the country can improve your chances of gaining a place.

Seeing how nursing numbers are generated

The provision of healthcare in the UK is an enormous business and it will continue to be a considerable employer of registered nurses for many years to come. Ensuring that there are enough nurses to cope with the ever-changing healthcare demands requires very intricate workforce planning.

The demand for NHS services is on the increase. With demographic changes such as an aging population, an increase in the public's expectations of quality care and advances in treatments, the National Audit Office predicts that growth in NHS activity is about 3 per cent per year. This growth in activity requires thoughtful planning, and when predicting how many nurses are needed in the future, the commissioning boards considers changes in health service delivery, the aging profile of nurses, the likely number who'll retire or leave, and the cost implications of educating new nurses.

Your local health boards or hospital trusts consider all the factors and decide how many nurses and from which nursing fields they will need in future years. They report their future nursing needs to their relevant commissioning boards. These are the organisations that consider the financial budgets and set the nursing numbers. It's these commissioning boards that tell the universities how many student nurse places they'll fund (different universities take on different numbers of students). Student numbers fluctuate against the changing healthcare requirements, and so some years you see a drop in overall numbers, but other years you see an increase. But if all works according to plan, by the time each nurse completes their education, a qualified nurse vacancy is available to fill.

The universities therefore have little say in the number of students they can recruit, and they receive the financial funding only for the agreed numbers. So no advantage exists in over-recruiting unless universities have arrangements in place to allow you to pay the full cost of your nurse education yourself (which is very expensive!).

Chapter 9

Making the Most of Open Days and Visits

. . . .

In This Chapter

▶ Researching and planning before your visit

▶ Getting the information you need from university staff

▶ Assessing the university

▶ Attending other university events

. . . .

*O*pen days are an excellent opportunity to get a feel of what universities have to offer and whether they are all that you imagined. Even after reading the prospectus from cover to cover you only know what the university wants you to know. It's not until you actually visit the university that you find out whether this is the place you want to spend the next three or four years.

You can't visit every university that offers your nursing field, but you can attend open days for those you most like the look of. Doing so helps you whittle down your choices to a shortlist and get a feel for which university you'd most like to attend.

You may have decided on your first choice of university already based on information you've read, and so you don't feel the need to attend an open day. My advice is to go and check out the campus in any case so that you're making an informed choice. At the least, you confirm you've chosen wisely, but you may just unearth a few aspects of university life that you hadn't considered.

This chapter offers useful hints to help you plan and make the most of your university visits.

Planning Prior to Your Visit

UCAS allows you to apply to up to five separate universities and so you need to decide if you visit each one or just a selection. This may well depend on the dates of the open days, the costs involved in attending each university or your availability and the convenience of attending. Plan to attend at least two open day events. No two universities are the same, and seeing more than one university allows you to compare and contrast what's on offer.

Your first job is to check the dates of open days. Each university has several throughout the year. They're normally timed to fit in with the UCAS cycle, giving you the chance to make your visit before sending off your application form. Different universities' open day dates may clash.

Many universities won't consider your application after 15 January. If you want to attend an open day before submitting then plan at least six months ahead. You can attend a July event in one year even though you're applying for nursing in October of the following year.

When you have a list of dates, plan what you want to see. Each university website provides detailed information on open days, with dedicated pages explaining what's on offer and a programme of events. Be sure to note which events require pre-booking, to avoid disappointment, and keep in mind that morning events are usually busier, so spread your events through the afternoon as well.

Here are aspects to explore at the university:

- ✔ **Central exhibition.** In central areas staff and students are on hand to offer advice about all aspects of the open day, not just nursing. Here you find lots of general information about the university and its facilities, and you pick up handouts and freebies. An ideal place to start your visit, especially if you're lost!

- ✔ **Drop-in sessions.** No need to book onto these sessions; staff and students are available to speak with you as you arrive at the venue. These sessions are good for individual queries you have about nursing and the programme.

- ✔ **Student life talks.** Look out for financial advice events where you can hear about money matters. Also take a wander around the students' union.

✔ **Subject talks.** Arranged at specific times throughout the day, these talks give a general overview of the nursing programme. Hearing about how the programme is organised and how you learn as a student is very useful. You can also meet the admissions team.

✔ **Taster lectures.** Many nursing departments use their clinical suites for these sessions, so you get a feel for the venue as well as an insight into how students are taught. You can often try your hand at a clinical skill. Booking is usually essential because spaces are limited.

✔ **Tours.** Student representatives show small groups of visitors around various parts of the campus. You usually find several options for tours, such as teaching facilities, sports department, catering areas or accommodation. Must-sees include first-year accommodation, clinical suites and the hospital. The library is another place to explore – you can usually do this without a tour guide.

Also make time to explore the local area. Consider amenities like supermarkets, accommodation, travel links and nightlife.

On the Day: Meeting Staff and Students

Good universities have an entire team to help with the open day. The team members have different roles and responsibilities, and their job is to answer your questions and give you a good sense of nursing department. Of course, they do their best to show you that the department is friendly and well organised.

In turn, while asking questions of departmental staff and students, you need to be making an effort to make a good impression. They want to appeal to the *best* students, and you want them to think that means you.

Knowing who's who

You have the opportunity to talk to the different members of the team, and each can help in different areas:

✔ **Admissions tutor:** Probably the most important person for you to see at the open day. Invariably, they're registered nurses and also lecturers with academic profiles, so they get involved with research and the teaching of nursing students. Often they also have a personal tutor role so they know a lot about how students cope on the programme. Admission tutors have a complete understanding of the admissions process and can help you with:

- Understanding entry grades and any alternatives.

- The UCAS process and dates you must work to.

- How to write your personal statement.

- Appreciating what's involved in the selection process.

- Understanding any selection assessments.

- Knowing how decisions are made.

✔ **Lecturers:** Many lecturers like to get involved with open days. They don't all have a great deal of knowledge about how admissions work, but they do have a wealth of knowledge about the nursing programme. A range of lecturers is often available, which may include the head of department or the clinical tutor, and all have experience teaching and supporting students. Lecturers are good to talk to when finding out about the learning opportunities and different experiences you can expect while on the programme. Lecturers can:

- Explain how your teaching is planned on a weekly basis.

- Discuss the different assessments you undertake during your studies.

- Show how the pastoral role works.

- Explain the level and type of supervision you can expect.

✔ **Student ambassadors:** Universities encourage students to get involved with open days because they often have the greatest impact on your opinions. Student ambassadors are carefully selected to give the right impression; however, more often than not they ask for the opportunity to be involved because they recognise the importance of selecting good future students. Ambassadors are experienced students who can give insight into the daily life of being a student nurse. They can:

- Answer those 'silly' questions that you don't want to ask the admissions tutor.

- Tell you how to save money, such as through car sharing.

- Explain what living in student accommodation is really like.

- Give you the lowdown on the quality of lectures and the level of support.

Making a good impression

A good impression means getting involved, asking appropriate questions, talking with various staff and showing a professional attitude. The day can be quite long, so wear clothes that are comfy and appropriate for the weather – but that also demonstrate your understanding of professionalism. A relaxed and casual approach without a heavy reliance on logos or distressed clothes is most suitable.

When meeting with university representatives, be sure to:

- ✔ **Attend talks and information sessions on time.** Staff will notice if you arrive late and interrupt the session as you take your seat.

- ✔ **Turn your mobile off or put it on silent.** A ringing phone is very distracting and people will think you're rude for leaving it on.

- ✔ **Keep any child you take with you under control.** A crying baby or noisy child attracts the wrong type of attention. If possible, take someone with you who can look after the child.

- ✔ **Do the talking yourself if you visit with parents.** Parents have good intentions and like to ensure you get the best information, but take the lead. Admissions tutors want to hear the questions from you.

- ✔ **If going as a group, be polite and not rowdy.** Have fun and enjoy the day, but don't upset other visitors or cause a commotion.

You have opportunities to ask questions, and doing so is a great way to get noticed. You could ask any of the following questions:

- ✔ What are the term dates? (Nursing students have a longer academic year.)

- ✔ What is the holiday entitlement? (It's less than for other university students.)

- ✔ How is clinical practice integrated into the programme?

- ✔ How does mentorship work with the programme?

- ✔ What unusual areas of clinical practice are available to students?

Only ask questions that haven't already been discussed. Repeating questions shows you haven't been listening or have missed the point.

Evaluating the University

Open days are long days, and after meeting many people, listening to lots of talks and visiting many departments, by the time you get home everything may become a blur. Make yourself a checklist to help you evaluate the day, grading elements of the university on a scale of 1 to 10. See Table 9-1 for an example.

Table 9-1	Open Day Evaluation			
Aspect	*University 1*	*University 2*	*University 3*	*University 4*
Campus				
Nursing department				
Nursing talk and tour				
Accommodation				
Catering facilities				
Library and IT services				
Clinical placements				
Clinical skills suite				

Don't be shy about taking pictures on the open day; most mobile phones take a picture quite discreetly. Pictures help remind you of the different places and departments you visited.

Plan to take someone with you on the day who can give a second opinion on the campus. Your friend or family member may see things you miss. Sit down together afterwards and compare notes on aspects of the university.

Taking Advantage of Other Visits and Tours

Open days are the universities' main events to advertise their campus and get you to consider their programmes and degrees. But universities run other smaller-scale events throughout the year.

Summer schools and taster courses

Many universities offer courses for candidates whose families have no experience of higher education. The intention is to offer first-hand experience of what it is to be a university student. You can take a course over the summer or as a taster:

- ✔ **Summer schools** can be residential as well as day-only programmes. Normally, candidates are still at school and have been offered places on the programme as part of the *Widening Participation* initiative, which helps students with good academic potential from lower social and economic backgrounds to experience university life.

- ✔ **Taster courses** are short programmes relating to nursing and healthcare subjects. They're normally open to Year 11 and 12 students, but universities do arrange similar events for mature students attending college. Taster courses offer an opportunity to see how the subjects that students are currently studying relate to higher education.

These events are directed at giving potential nursing students the chance to experience study at university and get involved with lectures, academic writing, presentations and teamwork. They're useful in helping you decide that university is for you, but they only offer limited support with regards to the application process.

Campus tours

If you can't make an open day then a campus tour might be sufficient to give you an impression of what student life is like at the university. Campus tours run frequently throughout the year and are open to all candidates and their parents or friends. These tours are student led, so you get the opportunity to speak with current students, although not necessarily nursing students.

Campus tours last only a few hours and consist of a tour around the main buildings such as the library, catering and sports facilities. They don't include viewing accommodation.

Campus tours don't routinely visit the nursing departments. If you want to speak with the nursing team or have a tour of the nursing department, you need to make contact with the nursing admissions team separate from your booking for the campus tour.

Applicant visit days

After you make your application and include a university as one of your choices, the university may invite you to an applicant visit day to persuade you to make it your first choice (or sometimes you can book a place yourself). Although applicant visit days aren't a substitute for open days, if you've been unable to visit the university, this is a great opportunity to meet the team and see the campus.

Plan to spend the whole day at the university, because there'll be a strict programme of events. On the day you can:

✓ Meet admission tutors and academic and clinical teams.

✓ Attend a talk on the university history, student services and financial support.

✓ Go to taster lectures and clinical skills sessions.

✓ Tour the campus, including all the main facilities such as the library and catering and sports facilities.

✓ Visit the nursing department.

✓ Visit the student accommodation.

Chapter 10

Money Matters

· ·

In This Chapter
▶ Adding up the costs of training to be a nurse
▶ Taking advantage of financial support
▶ Getting a job to ease the burden

· ·

*E*ducation is a costly business, and one of the main reasons that student nurses quit their programme is lack of finances. Many fail to appreciate how much money they need to manage their studies and meet their other commitments. Both your preparations to gain a place on a nursing programme and the course itself put a strain on your purse strings. Knowing this upfront and preparing for the impact that money (or the lack of) has during your time as a nursing student eases the hardship that finances can cause.

In this chapter, I explain the important aspects of financial planning. I give you insight into the costs of preparing yourself to apply to university, covering the bills for the application and the selection events. And I look closely at the various costs associated with being a nursing student, and how you can manage your money when you start on the programme.

Tallying the Costs of Your Education

In comparison to other university students, nursing students appear to have a good deal when it comes to financing their education. To undertake a non-healthcare degree requires a significant investment of £7–9,000 per year for course fees alone, and many students take on student maintenance loans that result in a substantial debt that takes a long time to repay once in employment. In comparison, student nurses don't have course fees to pay, and they can receive what some see as very generous rewards for going into nursing (see the later section 'Grants, loans and bursaries').

But don't fall into the trap of assuming that nursing is an inexpensive programme to follow. Preparing for nursing is a costly business. The following sections outline all the costs you can expect to cover when training to be a nurse.

Academic fees

Your aspirations to be a nurse can be quite expensive. Depending on the route you take to gain your qualifications, the financial cost can be a small fortune, made up of small, one-off payments such as for enrolment fees or administration costs, to substantial sums for course fees and assessments.

Gaining entry qualifications

Chapter 3 reviews the range of academic qualifications that support applications. The cost of gaining these entry qualifications depends on how you're studying:

- ✔ **Full-time.** If you're in school or college and yet to leave the education system, then the cost of your education is inexpensive. The government subsidises the course fees of students who are still in full-time education of more than 15 hours a week, which makes attending school or college relatively cheap. If you're returning to study as a mature student and take a full-time course, the costs vary depending on where you study and your eligibility for financial support. Some local colleges subsidise full time study over 15 hours a week and you pay nothing, while others can charge £500 for a full-time course.

- ✔ **Part-time.** If you plan to undertake your studies as a part-time student then you may have to pay the full costs for the teaching and assessments for your subjects. Generally studying part-time is more expensive because the subsidies to support you in your local college are less generous. You could be expected to pay up to £1,000 for a part-time course.

If you're returning to study as a mature student then consider the cost of each route in terms of managing your other commitments. Some mature students, for example, want to study part time to help manage their paid employment or for childcare reasons. But when offsetting the extra education costs against wages or childcare costs, becoming a full-time student may work out cheaper overall.

Most educational providers can arrange for you to pay in manageable instalments rather than one lump sum. Read the prospectus or contact the organisation directly for detailed information on payment methods.

Also factor in these related costs that you may incur while studying for your entry qualifications:

- ✔ Administrative fee for enrolment: £45–70

- ✔ Criminal Record Bureau (CRB) check (if your course has clinical placements): £44

- ✔ Books and study aids: At least £45

Paying for nursing programmes

All nursing programmes are supported by central government funding, which means the government pays your course fees directly to your university. You don't pay educational fees throughout the duration of the course.

However, the government has strict rules of eligibility that every nursing student has to meet in order to receive the fee waiver. To be eligible you must be able to demonstrate that you're a European Union citizen and have completed ten years formal education. Although all the countries of the UK have this broadly similar rule, check the rules for the specific country where you plan to study.

Many universities have limited places and can only support students who have eligibility for both course fees and bursary entitlement (see the section 'Grants, loans and bursaries', later in this chapter). Other universities accept students who receive fees-only awards. Double-check with your chosen university to avoid disappointment.

The cost of applying to university

The application process can be quite lengthy, and depending on the number of choices you make and where each university is in relation to home, you could spend a significant amount of money managing each of your choices before you make a final decision. Remember to include the actual cost of applying to university when you're calculating how much money you need to save. Consider some of these potential costs (correct at the time of writing):

✔ **Charge to UCAS for submitting application:** You pay an initial cost to apply (£12) and then an additional cost if you make more than one choice on your application form (£11). Using all five choices initially costs £23. If you apply late in the UCAS cycle, you may be charged a higher fee for a single-choice application (£23).

✔ **CRB check:** Although you may already have a CRB report from college or through work, universities usually require their own copies. Expect to pay for another enhanced CRB check (£44).

✔ **Legal and academic documents:** The university requires proof of your eligibility for funding. Do you have all the original documents necessary, such as your birth certificate, evidence of qualifications, any name-change deed and your driving licence? If you need duplicates, you have to pay for these, from £20 for a replacement driving licence, to £37 for replacement academic certificates.

✔ **Health check:** Universities undertake these on potential students. You may have to travel to the university for their own nurse to assess you, or your GP may be allowed to complete the check. Either way, you need to consider travel costs or GP expenses.

✔ **Travel:** You'll be travelling to universities for open days and applicant days (see Chapter 9) and interviews. You may need to arrive early, so consider arranging accommodation for the night before. And don't forget to add to the projected costs those coffees and sandwiches on campus.

✔ **Extra sundries:** Think about all those little extras that you may have to find money for. For example, do you need a new set of clothes to attend the interviews? Does the university expect you to print off documents to complete and return by post? Are you required to hand in photocopies of all your documents?

If you've been in care then speak with your chosen university about their care leavers support package. As part of their widening participation programmes, universities have finance available to help with open days and UCAS applications, and they offer support for all-year-round accommodation.

Clinical expenses

When you study on a nursing degree, not only do you have to cover the normal costs of being a student, but you have the added expense of the clinical aspect of the programme too.

Travel expenses

You attend clinical practice for at least 50 per cent of your degree programme. Patients are nursed in a variety of places and you are required to visit different locations. Depending on how your university plans clinical experiences, the distance you have to travel and the expense varies. Universities attempt wherever possible to consider your mode of transport and place of residence when arranging clinical placements, but do expect a lot of travelling.

If you're eligible to receive a bursary, you may claim some of your travel expenses back. Currently, if you travel five miles for study but need to get to a clinical placement nine miles away, you're able to claim for the extra four miles. This may be claimed as mileage if you use your own car or reimbursed if the bus or train fare is more than it costs to get to university. You must keep your receipts to claim. Also, if you're using your car to travel to a client's home in the community you must ensure that your car insurance covers you for this activity.

Equipment costs

Nursing is a professional and vocational programme, and you're required to be suitably equipped for the clinical part of the programme. Here are items you may have to pay for:

- ✔ **Documentation:** Some universities require you to pay for the files containing all the health and safety training and clinical assessments for the programme. If the university provides the documentation free of charge, you can expect to pay a charge for any replacements.

- ✔ **Identification badges:** Provided free initially but you pay for any replacements.

- ✔ **Medical kit:** Some nursing programmes require you to buy your own clinical equipment such as a face mask, stethoscope and scissors.

- ✔ **Nurse's watch:** You can't wear a normal wristwatch for clinical work as it's an infection risk. The popular alternative is to have a nurse's fob watch to wear on your uniform.

- ✔ **Nursing books:** Universities hold many of the necessary books in their libraries and give the reading lists of the essential textbooks. Be prepared to buy your own copies of some of the more popular books that are always on loan. Consider also subscribing to a nursing journal such as *Nursing Standard* or *Nursing Times*.

✓ **Uniforms:** Normally, the university covers the cost of uniforms, but you may be charged to replace items that are damaged, such as through shrinkage due to incorrect laundering.

Professional union fees

As a student working towards nurse registration you're treated differently to other university students. In particular, your clinical practice exposes you to public scrutiny and civil accountability, and the professional regulator (the NMC) requires a standard of performance and behaviour from you. So your university is likely to recommend that you're a member of a trade union.

UNISON (www.unison.org.uk/) is a popular option, but also consider the Royal College of Nursing (www.rcn.org.uk) as a suitable alternative due to its nursing emphasis. You pay a fee to join a trade union, but the rates are reduced for students and only cost £10 per year.

Housing considerations

For nursing students, the largest cost of attending university is undoubtedly the expense of having somewhere to live for the duration of the programme.

You may have the choice of living at home while you study. Many students choose this option if their university is within reasonable travelling distance. Living in the family home means that the typical housing costs, such as council tax, utility bills and food costs, are cheaper than student accommodation so you face negligible extra expense when attending university.

You may, however, not have the option to live at home, or choose to have the full student experience and move into student residence. In this case you have two choices:

✓ **University accommodation:** Universities offer first-year students accommodation in their own halls of residence (many universities expect students to move into rented housing for the remainder of their studies). The accommodation is either run by the university itself or in collaboration with a letting organisation, and you have a choice between self-catering or catered. If you apply late you may find that university accommodation isn't guaranteed.

✓ **Rented student accommodation:** Plenty of options are available for students who choose to live in rented accommodation, or who have to due to applying late or through clearing. Universities work with letting agencies and landlords to

Chapter 10: Money Matters **149**

ensure student receive the best deals, so discuss your accommodation needs with the university's accommodation office in the first instance rather than directly with an agency or private landlord. Check with your local council, as you may be able to receive a council tax subsidy while a student in rented accommodation.

Table 10-1 helps you compare the costs of the two kinds of accommodation.

Table 10-1   Comparing the Costs of University and Rented Accommodation

Cost	University Accommodation	Rented Accommodation
Administration fee	No	Payable when renting through an agency
Weekly rent	Higher	Lower
Deposit	Payable	Payable
Utility bills	Included	Payable
Internet access	Included (may be limited)	Not included
TV licence	Payable	Payable
Contents insurance	Included (but limited)	Payable
Furniture	Included	Often included (may be limited)
Contract period	42–45 weeks	52 weeks

All accommodation, whether university or private, requires an initial deposit (typically £250–500), which is only returned at the end of the contract. The deposit covers any damage to the accommodation, so be sure to leave your room in good repair.

When considering accommodation, also think about parking and travel costs. Living in a flat in the city that's a bus-ride from the university campus means you'll need a bus pass. Most accommodation has limited parking, and you may need to buy a permit, which can be quite expensive depending on the location of the accommodation.

Kitting yourself out for independent living

Living away from home means that you require everyday essentials that you need to budget for, although halls accommodation may be pretty well equipped. Here's a starting point for your list:

✔ Two sets of bed linen, blankets or duvet and maybe pillows.

✔ Iron, ironing board and coat hangers.

✔ Kitchen utensils such as cutlery, crockery and pots and pans.

✔ Pictures, posters and trinkets to decorate your room (check the halls contract, as not all allow you to hang pictures or posters on the wall).

✔ Extension leads (power sockets can be limited).

Depending on how well kitted out your accommodation is, you may also need furniture and electrical items like a kettle and toaster. But delay buying items such as irons, toasters and kettles until you arrive, because you may be able to share with other students.

Living expenses

The general cost of living can be very expensive, and it's often the small charges that add up to the biggest bills. Living on your own is more costly than sharing, so here's a 'budget' list of weekly essentials which of course can increase based on your own lifestyle!

Rent	£100
Food	£50
Gas and electricity	£15
Internet	£8
Mobile phone	£10
Laundry	£8
Clothes	£15
Travel (to university)	£13
Socialising	£20

And don't forget those 'one-off' bills…

TV licence	£145
Internet installation	£50
Student insurance	£110

Getting Financial Support

Reading the preceding section 'Tallying the Costs of Your Education' could make you feel demoralised about all the expense associated with being a nursing student. However, the news isn't all doom and gloom, because this section outlines ways in which you can reduce the cost of your education. The government, in particular, has many schemes that help cushion the costs of study.

 The following sections outline the financial support that may be available to you. Support is calculated against your personal and financial circumstances. Appreciate that funding levels change from student to student and not everybody receives the same level of assistance.

 Financial assistance is based on your individual circumstances, and those who make the assessments require very specific information from you. No information means no assistance. Plan ahead and collect all the necessary documents and information so that you receive your full entitlement.

Help with entry qualification costs

Depending on your circumstances, you may be able to receive financial assistance in covering the cost of your course or education prior to the nursing programme. Here's a selection of schemes that give an example of what's available:

- ✔ **Learning grant:** For those from low-income families. The money is intended to help cover the cost of study aids, books, travel and childcare while studying.

- ✔ **Enhanced Learning Credits Scheme (ELC):** This Ministry of Defence initiative provides funding to support members of the armed forces to study nationally recognised qualifications, which helps prepare them for new careers in civilian life.

- ✔ **Redundancy reaction schemes:** Directed at those under threat of redundancy or who've recently become unemployed. The intention is to remove barriers to employment by retraining and learning of new skills.

- ✔ **Higher Education Funding Council:** Offers receive financial assistance if you're on a low income for some part-time higher education courses offered at colleges.

- ✔ **Subsidised bus pass:** Many local education authorities offer bus travel at a reduced rate for students.

Grants, loans and bursaries

Not having to pay course fees on the nursing programme is a welcome relief, but you still need to support yourself – and if circumstances require it, your family and dependents – while undertaking
the nursing degree.

The NHS *bursary scheme* aims to provide financial support to a
wide range of NHS-funded courses that lead to a professional registration. The scheme is open to many healthcare students, not
just nursing students, and the intention is to ensure that the NHS
attracts high-calibre students from a diverse range of backgrounds.
The support provided is to cover the day-to-day living costs of
your study and any money is exempt from tax and national insurance contributions.

In order to be considered for assistance through the scheme you
must meet the eligibility criteria:

✓ **Personal eligibility:** You may not be considered for funding
   if you're financially supported by your current employer.
   Sometimes students are supported by their employer to
   undertake nurse training and continue to get their wage while
   doing so. In these cases, depending on the amount you earn,
   you may be disqualified from receiving the bursary.

✓ **Residential eligibility:** Regardless of your nationality, you
   must be resident within the UK for the three years up to the
   date that you start your course. What is classed as 'ordinarily
   residential' is quite complicated, so you need to be sure that
   you qualify. The following situations require further consideration by the bursary team who are assessing your application
   and you may be asked to provide more evidence of your resi-
   dency:

   • You're a UK citizen but work or live abroad.

   • You have refugee or migrant worker status.

   • You only have limited leave to remain in the UK.

   • The Home Office has made declarations regarding your
     settlement in the UK.

Understanding the rules and having the evidence in advance
speeds up your application for bursary. Don't be surprised just
how many documents and pieces of evidence are needed to complete your assessment. And because the income of your parent,
spouse or partner is taken into consideration, make sure they are
happy to provide the information. Without their assistance your
application may not succeed.

The bursary scheme consists of three elements: the grant, the bursary and the student loan. Each is assessed quite differently and you have to re-apply for financial assistance at the beginning of each academic year.

Grant

This is a set sum of £1,000 that's offered to all students regardless of their financial situation if offered an NHS funded nursing place. It's not means tested (see the next section) and you don't have to repay it at the end of the programme. The grant is usually paid into your bank account at intervals throughout the year rather than one lump sum.

Bursary

This is the largest component of the scheme, and the level of financial assistance you receive is based on your individual circumstances.

Means testing means that the bursary team considers the income from your parents, spouse or partner. Calculations are made against the income after tax, and your casual income while studying as a full-time student isn't normally taken into account.

If you live at home your parents' income is assessed; you won't receive a bursary without this assessment.

The means testing calculates how much those supporting you contribute to your bursary, and the higher the contribution, the lower the bursary. Contributions usually commence when after-tax income exceeds approximately £24,000. Table 10-2 gives an example.

Table 10-2	How Your Parents' Income Affects Your Bursary
Residual Income	**Bursary Reduced By**
Under £24,279	Nil
£24,279	£45
£25,000	£120
£27,500	£384
£30,000	£647
£32,500	£910

When calculating the level of bursary, the scheme considers whether you're an independent student (not reliant on your parents' income). To be independent you need to meet one of the following criteria:

- ✔ You have a dependent child.
- ✔ You're married.
- ✔ You've supported yourself for at least 36 months prior to starting the course.

The bursary team also takes into account other elements of your commitments and the programme in the means testing:

- ✔ **Where you study.** The basic bursary amount is more for the London region than elsewhere, but living in your parents' home gains a smaller allowance.
- ✔ **The length of the programme.** Additional weekly allowances are available should the programme run beyond 30 weeks.
- ✔ **Dependants.** You can claim a dependants allowance if people are wholly or mainly financially dependent upon you. You can also get assistance if you use registered childcare providers, and a parent learning allowance may be payable. Maternity pay can be paid as existing bursary should you find yourself pregnant while on the programme.
- ✔ **Travelling costs.** You can claim for the costs of travelling back and forth to your clinical placements (but not university). See the previous section 'Travel expenses'.
- ✔ **Disability.** The disabled students' allowance offers financial assistance to cover extra help to complete your course after you have the appropriate assessment of needs.

The NHS has a fraud department that investigates and prosecutes when fraudulent claims for student finance have been made. Make sure you provide accurate and truthful evidence when making your application. Making assumptions or miscalculations can land you in hot water!

Student loan

As part of the bursary scheme you're eligible to apply for a reduced-rate student loan. This is a maintenance loan because the bursary doesn't cover all your living costs. The loan is means tested and is repayable. You have to repay the loan after you commence paid employment and reach a certain annual income, currently in excess of £21,000, which starts after you've been working for a full year. The sum repaid each month is deducted by your employer.

You make applications for the loan separately to the bursary application, and doing so is totally optional: you don't need to apply should you be able to balance your finances. Here's an example of the loans available:

- ✔ Living away from home: £2,324
- ✔ Living at home: £1,744

You make the application to your country's student loan company. To find which organisation you need to apply to for your student loan, search the UCAS student finance page at `www.ucas.ac.uk/students/studentfinance/`. It gives useful information and tells you where to go for the right advice.

 Students are good at applying for the bursary but forget that the student loan requires a separate application to a different organisation. A delay in applying results in a delay receiving your money.

Scholarships

Scholarships are a popular way for universities to attract the better students. The university offers the scholarship to entice candidates to choose this university over other options. Most scholarships award money as a gift (not to be repaid) to cover course fees or as a contribution to living expenses. The successful student has to meet the eligibility criteria. For example, students may need to achieve specific academic grades or commit to excelling in a particular sport.

The problem for you is that student nurses rarely meet the eligibility criteria for a scholarship. Receiving an NHS bursary in most cases exempts you from applying for scholarships supporting living costs, and not having to pay course fees means those scholarships aren't relevant either!

Still, look at the information of your chosen university to see what is on offer and whether you can apply. Two common scholarships may be available to you:

- ✔ **Excellence scholarship:** Awarded to students who achieve high grades in the pre-entry qualifications. If you're predicted to achieve A and B or equivalent grades then it's worth investigating whether you could apply for this award.
- ✔ **Sports Scholarship:** Are you a keen sportsperson and achieving to a distinguished level? If so your university may consider offering financial support if you continue your sporting activities at the university.

A few external organisations offer scholarships to nursing students. These awards are usually to help with attending conferences or undertaking research, but they could be useful in supporting your studies. Examples include:

- ✔ **The Cavell Nurses' Trust Scholarships** offer awards up to £2,000 to help student nurses with the expenses incurred when working in tailor-made clinical placements. This money is helpful if you want to experience a particular type of nursing that your university doesn't normally offer and you have to contribute to the costs. The Trust also offers scholarships of £1,500 to student nurses who excel in their passion for nursing. The award is offered to those students demonstrating commitment and professionalism to nursing.

- ✔ **The Royal College of Nursing Margaret Parkinson Scholarship** is a specific award of up to £2,000 for people who already hold a degree and wish to train as a nurse. There is no requirement on how the scholarship is spent, but you are required to attain a certain academic level during the course.

Tax allowances

A student nurse in full-time education can benefit from certain tax allowances. Taxes are assessed against your specific circumstances and so you may not be eligible for all the benefits. Check with your local authority or Jobcentre Plus to enquire about your eligibility for:

- ✔ Child tax credit
- ✔ Council tax benefit
- ✔ Housing benefit
- ✔ Social security benefits
- ✔ Working tax credits

Hardship funds

Universities have contingency funds to support students who get into financial difficulty. These plans have money set aside to help students in adversity, but the funds are limited and you must meet strict criteria to receive help. The university assesses your needs, and, if you qualify, you receive a one-off payment.

Examples of when these funds would not be granted are for the purchase of books or to help with travel costs.

REMEMBER

Hardships funds are there to help with unforeseeable expenses such as costs for disability assessments or breakdown of your PC, and you should use them as the last resort, when you've exhausted all other options.

Tips on managing money

- Buy a student railcard or bus pass.

- Use your student union card to get discounts in shops and food halls.

- Use the university sports centre – it could be cheaper than the local gym.

- Pack your own lunch or use the university's meal plan – or visit `my supermarket.co.uk` and `supermarketownbrandguide.co.uk` for money-saving tips.

- Buy second-hand books. Try CheapUniBooks (`http://cheapunibooks. co.uk`). Other students may be able to loan or sell their books to you if they've completed part of the course.

- Don't use pay-day loans; the annual percentage rate (APR) is expensive.

- Get a student bank account with agreed overdraft facilities.

- Visit the university money advice website for local help and tips.

- Be prepared to share a bathroom; it's a lot cheaper than having an en suite room.

- Not good with your money? Use Money Supermarket for tips and advice (`www. moneysupermarket.com`).

Part IV

Perfecting Your Application

Top Five Tips on Submitting Your Personal Statement

- ✔ Use up to 4,000 characters and no more in your statement. Characters are each individual letter, digit or space and not individual words.

- ✔ Use no more than 47 lines in your statement, which includes any line spaces.

- ✔ Don't use italics, bold script or underlined words. Such formatting is removed automatically, which may change the emphasis you hoped to make.

- ✔ Use ordinary keyboard characters. UCAS makes slight alterations to your statement if you insert certain characters. Double-check which ones are accepted and which ones are substituted if using European characters.

- ✔ Submit your statement once only. This statement has to cover all your choices and includes UCAS Extra.

Go to www.dummies.com/extras/getintonursing schooluk for free online bonus content created especially for this book.

In this part . . .

✔ Use UCAS to complete your nursing application, and know the submission dates you need to stick to.

✔ Write the best personal statement you can, to impress the admissions tutors.

✔ Avoid common pitfalls with your personal statement.

✔ Rustle up a wonderful reference from your tutor or employer to support your application.

Chapter 11

Following the UCAS Process

. . . .

. . . .

*A*ll nursing programmes are at degree level, and you follow a formal application process through the Universities and Colleges Admissions Service (UCAS). In this chapter, I explain how to use the UCAS system, identifying the different sections and explaining what to consider to ensure a trouble-free application.

Understanding UCAS

UCAS manages applications to all higher education courses in the UK. It's registered as a charity, so it works independently of government or university control. However, because of its importance with managing applications to higher education, it has close working relationships with schools and colleges, universities and the Department for Education.

Managing the application process is very busy work, and UCAS processes over 2.8 million applications from 700,000 students each year.

Don't think of UCAS merely as an obscure system to manage your application to university, but see it as a helpful friend who supports you through a stressful and complicated process, offering advice and guidance along the way.

UCAS is primarily a web-based organisation, and it's very interactive and user friendly. Designed with students in mind, the way it uses the latest technology makes it easy to navigate its website and simple to find the information you're looking for. Visit www.ucas.ac.uk and browse through the site, using the headings at the bottom of the page.

Making use of other UCAS websites

Be sure to check out these websites run by UCAS:

✔ **UCASConnect** (www.ucasconnect.com/): A multimedia service to help answer all your questions. Not only does it have its own website, but it uses social media sites such as Facebook, Twitter, Google+, LinkedIn and YouTube to connect with students. The site has bloggers who write interesting articles about daily application issues. The bloggers are parents, applicants, first-year students and UCAS advisors, so you get information from all those involved with actually applying.

✔ **YouGo** (www.ucas.com/yougo/): This is a UCAS-run community website for all prospective students. When you register with the site you have access to other applicants and are able to talk with other nursing students. You can talk with students who've gained places on the same course in the same university as you and can start making joint plans for when you start your programme . . . great for working out who brings the toaster and who gets the kettle!

✔ **UCASTV** (www.ucas.tv): The UCAS website dedicated to 'how-to' videos that offer advice on all aspects of the application process. The videos highlight useful tips and hints on how to manage your application and start university in the best way possible.

UCAS isn't exclusive to students, and sections of the website support parents, career advisors and also school, college and university staff.

Mapping Out the Application Process

Applying to university is a lengthy process, so be prepared to spend many months researching the universities, whittling down the options and planning your application. The application process is structured with specific instructions and dates. Understanding the process and planning to meet the deadlines make your experience less stressful and more manageable.

When to apply: The dates you need to know

UCAS has a calendar of dates throughout the year by which you and your chosen universities need to take action and make responses. The exact dates change slightly year on year, but are broadly similar. Here's a condensed version of the dates for UCAS applications:

15 September	The earliest date you can send your application to UCAS.
Mid-December	Universities start inviting candidates to interview.
15 January	Deadline date for UCAS to receive your application. The course might not be available or the university might not accept your application after this date.
5 February	If you've used all your choices (maximum of five) and have received no offers by this date, you can have an attempt through *UCAS Extra*.
1 March	Last date for universities to make their decisions if your application was received by 15 January.
8 May	You must make a decision by now on any offers if your application was sent before 15 January.
27 June	You need to reply to any offers by now if your application was sent after 15 January.
30 June	Last date for UCAS to receive your application (if you apply after this date you're deemed as a clearing application).
18 July	The last date by which the university makes a decision on your application.
25 July	You decide which offers to accept by this date.
Mid-August	Your academic results are released and your chosen university confirms the offer. Clearing opens if you did not meet the terms of your offer.
30 September	Clearing closes. If you don't have an offer by now you need to contact universities directly or re-apply for the following year.

Many universities won't accept applications after 15 January. It is at their discretion to consider applications after this date, so don't get caught out: apply early.

If you don't make a decision on any offers by the set date then UCAS will reject the place by default and you'll lose that offer.

How to apply: Organising your application

Applying to UCAS is only possible online. The UCAS system stores your application details and so you can apply from any place that has internet access.

You use two systems during the application process:

✔ **UCAS Apply:** You use this system to develop your application. You work your way through the application form and there are help points along the way to explain what information is needed. There are six sections to complete:

   • Personal details

   • Additional information

   • Course choices

   • Academic qualifications

   • Employment details

   • Personal statement and references

✔ **UCAS Track:** Allows you to follow the progress of your application. You automatically receive a link to Track after you submit your application and receive your welcome letter from UCAS confirming receipt of your application. The admissions tutor also has access to UCAS tracker and can see which applicants have responded to offers.

Payment is required before you can submit your application. The most it costs is £23 if you use all five choices.

Here are some tips on organising your application:

✔ You have up to five choices, but you don't need to use them all at once. You can add choices at a later date.

✔ If in school or college, use their centre for submitting your application, because then your tutor can monitor your application. Remember, to make the link you need their *buzzword* (a phrase or word that your school or college has set up in UCAS so you can link your application to your college or school's UCAS profile).

Providing the right information

UCAS uses software to detect fraud and cancels an application that contains false and misleading information. Chapter 4 explains the requirements for declaring criminal convictions and disabilities and Chapter 12 tells you about UCAS's similarity detection software, which weeds out plagiarism in applications.

✔ When completing the form, nominate a parent or spouse to have access to your account. This helps if actions are needed when you are away, such as on holiday. However, your parents or spouse can't discuss your application with the admissions tutor as this is protected by the data protection act.

✔ Have your application ready early so that your referee has time to attach his statement (see Chapter 13). UCAS becomes much busier the closer to deadline dates.

Managing Rejections

After he receives your application, the admissions tutor either rejects your application or invites you to interview. After interview, the tutor decides to reject your application or make you an offer. So you could face rejection at either of two points in the process.

If you get one rejection, don't panic. You hopefully have other choices that may accept you, so sit tight for now.

Unfortunately, sometimes all five choices reject you. This can be quite depressing, but it's not the end of the world. If possible ask each university for some feedback to find out why you were unsuccessful, because this information helps in the next part of the process.

When you haven't been offered a place, all isn't lost. You have two options to explore: UCAS Extra and clearing.

Using UCAS Extra: Having the extra choice

UCAS *Extra* is the part of the process that allows you to have additional attempts at gaining an offer of a place. You can apply to additional universities but can't re-apply to any of your initial choices. Here's what you need to know about Extra:

✔ You need to have used all of your five choices to be eligible to use Extra. The Extra icon appears in your choices section of UCAS Track if this option is available to you. The icon appears once all your five choices have been used; this might happen at different times to other candidates rather than at set dates.

✔ The admissions tutor will be aware that this is an extra choice and may ask why you have not been successful in your previous applications or interviews.

✔ You can apply to several universities through Extra, but only one at a time.

✔ You can't change your personal statement when using Extra, so think this through when writing your statement (see Chapter 12). The chances of gaining a place in adult nursing are quite slim if your personal statement is all about midwifery.

✔ If you don't secure a place in Extra, you automatically become eligible for clearing when you receive your exam results (see the next section).

Going into clearing: Seeking those unfilled places

Clearing is the system that allows you to apply for any university places that are still vacant. Although clearing becomes available to candidates from mid-July, the busiest time is after the exams results are published mid-August. Clearing is quite a frenetic time, and although UCAS displays those universities that are using clearing, you have to make contact with them individually and not through UCAS. Be prepared to make several phone calls as clearing gets extremely busy!

The admissions tutor discusses your application with you, normally over the phone and, if satisfied, makes a verbal offer. You then use the clearing choice in the Track section of your account to confirm the offer.

Consider clearing if:

✔ You have no offers after using your five choices and UCAS Extra.

✔ Your exam results were worse than expected and your university hasn't confirmed its offer to you.

✔ You didn't meet the terms of your insurance offer (see the next section) and have been rejected.

Receiving Offers

Fortunately, making decisions on offers is much simpler than managing rejections. Hopefully, you've succeeded in gaining several offers, which may cause a dilemma over which one to choose. Head to Chapter 17 for all the information on reviewing your options.

Chapter 12

Writing Your Personal Statement

*A*t the centre of every successful application is a great personal statement. This is your opportunity to shine and show the admissions tutor that you have what it takes to be a nurse. Your mission is to:

✔ Tell the admissions tutor why they should choose you over the other candidates.

✔ Explain to the admissions tutor how you are most suited for the nursing programme.

✔ Show your commitment to and enthusiasm for nursing.

Your personal statement is hugely important in your application because it can be the deciding factor between rejection and the offer of an interview. Unlike many other degree programmes, where the offer of a place is based purely on what is written in the application form (and your academic qualifications), with nursing there is an additional layer of assessment: all candidates provisionally offered a place on the nursing programme have a face-to-face meeting with the admissions team.

In the interview, the admissions tutor uses the personal statement as a basis for asking questions about your suitability for their programme and examines quite closely what you wrote and how you behave against what your wrote. They can base their final decision to offer a place on how accurate and authentic your personal statement is in relation to how you present yourself in person.

In this chapter, I show you how to write a great statement. By the end of this chapter you'll know what mistakes to avoid and you'll have plenty of ideas for how to shape a statement that impresses the admissions tutor.

Understanding the Rules

When submitting your application you must make sure it meets all the necessary requirements, both of the Universities and Colleges Admissions Service (UCAS) and the universities that you are applying to. Any discrepancies show up and demonstrate that either you didn't understand what's expected of you or that you're just careless in your attention to detail; both are poor reflections and can lead to a rejected application.

UCAS is very strict about what you can and can't do when it comes to submitting your statement. It receives thousands of statements each year and treats each application objectively and fairly. It can't make allowances for you making mistakes.

Here are the basic rules for submitting your statement:

- ✔ Use up to 4,000 characters and no more in your statement. Characters are each individual letter, digit or space and not individual words.

- ✔ Use no more than 47 lines in your statement, which includes any line spaces.

- ✔ Don't use italics, bold script or underlined words. Such formatting is removed automatically, which may change the emphasis you hoped to make. So, for example, if you're writing about the book *Jane Eyre*, format it 'Jane Eyre' rather than using italics.

- ✔ Use ordinary keyboard characters. UCAS makes slight alterations to your statement if you insert certain characters. Double-check which ones are accepted and which ones are substituted if using European characters.

- ✔ Write in either English or Welsh.

- ✔ Submit your statement once only. This statement has to cover all your choices and includes UCAS Extra (see Chapter 11).

A 'timed out' facility on the UCAS website closes the webpage after 35 minutes of inactivity. Use the Save button frequently so you don't lose your work.

If you exceed the character or line allocation your statement stops at that point. Don't submit an incomplete statement that stops mid-sentence! Admission tutors see this as a poor reflection of your ability to follow guidelines.

The Apply section of the UCAS website (see Chapter 11) offers some useful tips on how to write your personal statement, including some do's and don'ts and information on size and presentation.

Also check the websites of your chosen universities for hints on what is expected in a personal statement – both the general university-wide guidance and that which is specific to the nursing programme. Some state quite clearly what they want to see and how you need to write your statement, and others are more subtle in describing what they expect from candidates. Open days are also good opportunities to find out about what each university wants (head to Chapter 9 for more on university visits).

Looking at What You Include

Getting the content of your statement just right is not going to happen on your first draft, so don't expect an hour in front of the computer is all you need. You'll write many drafts before you're happy with the final version, and each draft is going to slightly change the emphasis of your work.

Start your statement plan early, leaving plenty of time for several drafts. UCAS has a flow chart (at www.ucas.ac.uk/students/ applying/howtoapply/personalstatement/) that helpfully illustrates a timeline for completing your statement, and it suggests planning three months before submission.

The following guidelines help you determine what to write in the statement.

Selecting information

You only have 4,000 characters with which to sell yourself; this doesn't equate to many words. Use the available space to your best advantage.

Distinguish between what you must include and what you would like to include, and don't bore the reader with irrelevant information. Does telling the admissions tutor that you had an operation 12 years ago really add substance to your statement? Ask yourself how each sentence supports your application.

Your UCAS application has sections for completed and current qualifications, so you don't need to replicate that information in your personal statement. However, if it isn't clear how you meet the entry qualifications then you may need to offer some explanation; for example, you want to use your human science module from your BTEC course as an alternative to GCSE science.

Don't mention any university names, even if you're only applying to one choice. If you don't receive any offers then you can use your statement for UCAS Extra or clearing (see Chapter 11).

Sharing your own ideas only

While you're preparing your statement you undoubtedly do a lot of investigating on the topic. Your school and college tutors offer advice, your friends come up with some great ideas and your parents have some thoughts on what you should or shouldn't include. Alongside these friendly, helpful hints you also look at numerous websites that offer examples of statements that you can download and use as templates for your own statement.

Nothing's wrong with seeking out all this help and using other people's ideas to direct and support the way in which you develop your statement. However, always keep in mind that your statement must be an accurate and factual account of your *own* thoughts, experiences and opinions.

It's easy to read so much information that eventually you can't remember if your final draft is all your own work or that of others. UCAS use similarity software that can detect the copying of work already submitted or used elsewhere. Each year they identify over 30,000 candidates who *plagiarise*; using other people's information as their own. If your work appears to resemble other statements then your chosen universities are informed and they'll decide whether to have you write a new statement or to reject your application.

Remember, if the university expects you to complete a literacy test they can use it to compare your writing style with the personal statement and see if the statement isn't all your own work.

Being truthful

Be honest in your statement. Admission tutors often use personal statements as a basis for the questions they ask you at interview, and they expect you to be able to discuss in detail anything you've written. Table 12-1 shows some examples when the candidate doesn't quite live up to expectations at interview.

Table 12-1	Examples of Exaggeration
The Exaggeration	*The Truth Revealed at Interview*
'Nursing is a long-time passion of mine and I am highly motivated and committed to becoming a nurse.'	The candidate has worked in retail for many years and was recently made redundant. She has never demonstrated an interest in healthcare work and knows little of what nursing is. Her motivation appears to be the bursary and paid course fees.
'I have vast experience of team-work and leadership, taking charge of groups, managing tasks and supporting others.'	The candidate has been a Girl Guide for two years, but not in the role of leader.
'I have experienced many nursing situations and looked after patients with a variety of illnesses.'	She worked as a volunteer in a hospital. She watched nurses but was not involved with the nursing care.

Using experiences to show key skills and qualities

Remember, the title of this part of the application is *personal* statement, so bring in personal experiences. Think about experiences from your personal life, school or college and employment and how they demonstrate the skills and attributes you have that support your application.

It's not all about you . . .

The admissions tutor sees thousands of statements in which candidates say why they want to be a nurse and what they hope to gain from nursing, and then they offer personal experiences to prove their point. But what the admissions tutor most wants to see is what you bring to the nursing profession; how your experiences show that you have something special to offer nursing; and what *patients* would gain from you becoming a nurse. So for each paragraph you write, ask yourself: 'What does this mean for nursing?'

An *ordinary* personal statement tells the admissions tutor about your desire to become a nurse, gives a few examples of how you have prepared yourself to apply and explains some experiences. This offers some insight into who you are, which is fine, but dull and mediocre.

An *excellent* personal statement discusses how you have used experiences to develop yourself to match the desired qualities of the student nurse.

Chapter 5 details the people skills that nurses need to have. Also think about the nursing programme itself. How can you demonstrate your ability to study at degree level? Here are a few skills and attributes to consider matching to your experiences:

- Care and compassion
- Organisation
- Problem solving
- Self-motivation
- Teamwork
- Using your own initiative
- Working to deadlines

Using work experience

Look for the transferable skills. Working on the checkout in the local supermarket might not sound a good job to support your application, but you can use the experience to show your numeracy, customer care and negotiation skills. Having a job in a call centre for an insurance company may sound light years away from nursing, but both require a well-developed telephone manner, refined oral skills, the ability to recall information and deal with difficult people.

A note on hobbies

You may like to include some hobbies or social activities in your personal statement to demonstrate breadth of abilities and that you're a rounded individual. Think seriously about the impression that such activities will have upon the admissions tutor.

For example, say you write that you read ten books a week. The tutor may take that to mean that you like to broaden your mind, or that you prefer to be alone than with people (not ideal for nursing). If you list plenty of 'out with friends' activities, the tutor may think you're good at maintaining relationships, or she may think you're more interested in socialising than work and study.

Here's an example of how to turn an unrelated work experience into a comparative assessment of your skills:

> **Before:** 'I work as a shop assistant for a high street clothes store. I enjoy speaking with the customers and helping them with their enquiries. On occasion I am put in charge of the changing facilities or shoe department.'

> **After:** 'I work for a high street clothes retailer. My role varies, which has helped my ability to be flexible in my work routine. Working alongside others has developed my teamwork skills, and I have learnt how to be accommodating and supporting of others to ensure work is completed well and on time. Importantly, I have to interact with customers and appreciate how good communication skills can produce positive experiences and prevent problems arising. I see these as essential skills needed in nursing.'

Incorporating care experience

Personal experiences that relate to care, such as being a patient or observing care given to a family member, can be an excellent way to develop your statement. Chapter 6 is all about gaining care experience. But do make sure you can closely relate experiences to the nursing profession.

Being a care assistant on a busy hospital ward, for example, sounds like the ideal experience. But don't be complacent and expect the reader to assume you understand nursing. Show you know that experience of one clinical area doesn't demonstrate all that is nursing, and that roles and responsibilities could be different from that of a student nurse.

Thinking about How You Write

How you write your statement is just as important as the information that you put into it. If you have some good experiences that demonstrate you're the ideal candidate, why spoil your chances with poor presentation of the facts? A well-written statement speaks volumes not only about your academic ability but also your attitude towards detail and your judgement on what's important.

Don't write your statement on your own. Get help and have someone read through and make comments. What makes sense to you may not make sense to others. A critical eye is invaluable.

Keeping the audience in mind

Remember who's going to read the statement. You're not writing a nursing essay for your tutor or putting together a CV for a job. Your statement is read by highly skilled and experienced admission teams. These teams have read thousands of statements, they have expectations of what they want to read in a statement and, more importantly, want they *don't* want to read.

Admission tutors are university lecturers and professors, so make your statement academically creditable. The reader is knowledgeable, so assume they understand nursing better than you. And be original. Avoid tired clichés and don't write the obvious; try to make your statement stand out.

Also make sure you have the tone right. This is a formal piece of writing, so avoid:

- **Colloquialisms:** For example, write 'anybody can care', not 'anyone can care'; 'I know with certainty', not 'I know for sure'; and 'I received an A grade', not 'I got an A grade'. Avoid slang and abbreviations.

- **Contractions:** So write *cannot*, not *can't*; *I have*, not *I've*; and *they will*, not *they've*.

Start your sentences off well without using *and*, *so*, *but* and *or*.

Structuring carefully

The flow and logical sequence of your statement is important. A sound logical structure helps you effectively convey your opinions and reasoning, but a haphazard approach leads to a jumbled and confused set of views that are difficult to follow. Remember, you want to encourage the admissions tutor to continue reading your statement and by the end fully understand who you are and what potential you have to be a nurse.

Think about the overall structure – introduction, main body and conclusion – and also the structure at a line-by-line level. Make sure sentences and paragraphs move naturally from one theme to the next. Lead your reader through your statement.

If you're not too sure how to get started with the structure of your personal statement, the mind map tool on the UCAS website (www. ucas.ac.uk/documents/statement/mindmap_mono.pdf) gives some good illustrations of how to structure your thoughts and ideas.

Making the most of every word

Think quality, not quantity. Have a short statement that delivers a punchy and exciting description of you rather than labouring on to the end with a dull and dreary account of recent work experience.

Be clear. The admissions tutor should be able to read from start to end and be left with an impression that you can construct a good discussion. She shouldn't be struggling to understand the meaning of some sentences or paragraphs. Avoid generalisations and vague expressions:

- ✔ 'I have been interested in nursing all my life. . . .' What does 'all' mean?

- ✔ 'I think hand-washing is a really important issue. . . .' Which aspects of hand-washing? Why?

- ✔ 'I feel that psychology is fundamental to nursing. . . .' Why?

- ✔ 'To be a good nurse you need communication and teamwork skills. . . .' So, do you have them?

- ✔ 'Research is important to help us understand lots of nursing issues. . . .' Do you have any examples?

Starting with a yawn . . .

You want to open your statement with a memorable sentence that makes the admissions tutor want to read on. You don't want to bore the tutor by using the following kinds of overused opening sentences:

- ✔ 'I am currently studying a BTEC National Diploma in Health and Social Care. . . .'

- ✔ 'Florence Nightingale once said, "The very first requirement in a hospital is that it should do the sick no harm." . . .'

- ✔ 'From a young age I have wanted to be a nurse. . . .'

- ✔ 'Nursing is a very challenging and demanding career. . . .'

- ✔ 'Ever since dressing up as a nurse when I was a child. . . .'

Although you want to show your enthusiasm for nursing, don't get carried away and use exaggerated language:

- ✔ Nursing is *amazing*. . . .

- ✔ Caring for children is *fantastic*. . . .

- ✔ The programme on offer gives you an *incredible* opportunity. . . .

- ✔ The human mind is *unbelievably* interesting. . . .

Proofreading to weed out mistakes

When you're happy with the writing, you need to go through with a fine-tooth comb and check the grammar, spelling and punctuation:

- ✔ Use uppercase letters appropriately: for example, use a capital letter at the beginning of a sentence and use 'I', not 'i', when writing about yourself.

- ✔ Make sure your sentences make sense. 'Here I show qualities of me is good at nursing' is not a good sentence; however, 'The qualities I describe here help demonstrate my suitability for nursing' works well.

- ✔ Use punctuation correctly, especially commas, apostrophes and full stops. These are the usual culprits in poor statements.

- ✔ Make sure your paragraphs are correct. One large paragraph or many one-sentence paragraphs read poorly. Have several paragraphs, each with its own subject and made up of several sentences.

When you've completed your statement put it aside for a few days. This helps clear your head, and when you return to it you're refreshed and able to see any mistakes. Alternatively, give it to someone else to proofread. They can read it objectively and point out any problems or mistakes that you missed.

Use a word processor to develop your statement and then cut and paste your final draft into your UCAS account. (Remember to check character numbers as they can differ between each system.) Then you can make use of the spellcheck on your computer. But remember that it's no substitute for checking your writing thoroughly. Common errors to watch for include *where* when you mean *were*, *their* when you mean *there* and *hear* when you mean *here*.

Avoiding Pitfalls

There are many reasons that you can fail to get that offer of an interview. Here are common reasons for rejection based on the personal statement and how you can avoid getting rejected for each:

- ✔ **You've chosen different fields of nursing, and you've made reference to each in your statement.** Making applications to more than one field causes difficulty in demonstrating your commitment to each of the fields in one statement. Either you focus too much on one field or you're so generalised that you fail to address the specific interest in any field. *To avoid:* write your statement in relation to the qualities that you have that are important for nursing such as the ability to empathise, communication skills or ability to manage difficult situations.

- ✔ **You've chosen one field of nursing but referenced care experiences for another field.** For example, you may have gained care experience in adult nursing but are applying for learning disabilities. In discussing your experiences you don't relate how they support your application but leave it for the admissions tutor to make assumptions. *To avoid:* Show which skills are transferable between fields and focus on one qualification at a time.

- ✔ **You fail to demonstrate sufficient knowledge about the nursing programme in your statement.** The admissions tutor expects you to understand that nursing is distinctly different to other university courses and that you have extra requirements such as clinical practice and professional behaviour to consider. *To avoid:* Give an indication that you understand that nursing requires clinical work as well as academic, or that you expect to work unsocial hours.

- ✔ **You don't develop your discussion and opinions in enough depth.** Competition is tough. Although you may have produced a good statement, it wasn't as strong as other applicants'. *To avoid:* Add details to support your opinions. Don't just say you're good at communicating with children; explain a situation that demonstrates this. If you say that nurses are the most important professionals in the healthcare team, back up your opinion with an explanation.

Chapter 13

Finding Solid References

• •

In This Chapter
▶ Finding the best referee
▶ Seeing what goes into a reference
▶ Taking charge of the process

• •

*T*he references section of the application form requires serious attention. You write every part of the application other than the references section. As honest as you are (see Chapter 12 for a warning on not being truthful), sometimes you may exaggerate your potential. So the admissions tutor uses the reference to gauge the accuracy of your application and consider whether to call you to interview or not. Your choice of referee has a significant impact on the impression that the admissions tutor has of you.

In this chapter, I help you understand the reference aspect of the application and I look closely at what references you need and what they cover. I also help you select the best person to be your referee, to give your application the best possible chance of success.

Deciding Who to Ask For a Reference

Universities offer some advice on whom they expect to be a referee. They give you advice during the application process, usually when they invite you to interview. The Universities and Colleges Admissions Service (UCAS – see Chapter 11) also offers help with your choices, which you can find on their website. But ultimately, you have to decide which person is going to make your application stronger.

The most important factor in choosing your referees is making sure you pick the right person for the job. You need someone you've been in contact with in the last year and who's known you for at least a year (some universities make this a rule).

A good referee:

- ✔ Supports the good things you say about yourself.
- ✔ Reinforces the positive behaviours and attitudes you highlight.
- ✔ Includes aspects of your character that you hadn't thought about.
- ✔ Adds credibility to your application.

In most cases the reference attached to your UCAS form is an academic reference that demonstrates your potential to do well studying on the nursing programme. It does give some insight into your character and suitability for nursing, but this part is often very limited.

The NMC requires all nursing students to have been assessed as having good character and expects universities to take into consideration your conduct, behaviour and attitude when making their decision about your application. Therefore, universities frequently ask for one or two more references to review your professional characteristics – your potential to be a good nurse.

Some universities ask for three references in total:

- ✔ An academic reference demonstrating your study skills.
- ✔ A job reference illustrating your work ethos.
- ✔ A character reference identifying your caring characteristics.

Your academic tutor

If you're currently studying, ask your tutor to be your referee. Normally, your school or college links your application form to its UCAS account so tutors can easily upload references. The references can include some organisational details about the subjects you're studying and provide some of the following information on you:

- ✔ An account of your performance in each of your subjects.
- ✔ Areas in which you excel.
- ✔ Demonstration of your motivation towards study.
- ✔ Your attendance levels.
- ✔ Your predicted and actual grades.
- ✔ Your relationship with teachers and other students.

If you're no longer in education and need to provide an academic reference, carefully consider your options.

If you left school or college recently, your tutor is ideal – he can easily write a reference for you using the organisation's link to UCAS even though you're an independent applicant.

If you haven't been in formal education for some time, consider how informal education may help you meet this request. Consider any short courses that include using study skills and any occupational training such as NVQ/SVQs.

Your employer

Your current employer is going to be top of the list when it comes to references. Undoubtedly, the university, when requesting an employer reference, will expect the most recent employer from your employment history except in situations where:

✓ You've been employed by them for a short period of time.

✓ A previous employer is more appropriate for nursing.

When considering employer references, think carefully about the impression it gives of you. Having a reference from a former manager and not from your current employer could raise suspicions that you're hiding a problem.

Depending on the size and nature of your employer, it may have set policies on managing references, and this could cause some difficulties for you.

Should your employer be happy to write an individual reference for you, expect to see details such as:

✓ Any disciplinary measures

✓ Attitude and commitment to the job

✓ Length of time with the employer

✓ Punctuality and periods of absence

✓ Reasons for leaving

✓ Role and responsibilities

✓ Teamwork abilities

But if your employer is a large national organisation, it is likely that it has a policy of not supplying individual references and only providing the basic details on:

- ✔ Confirmation of your employment
- ✔ Dates of your employment
- ✔ Your role in the organisation

This type of reference is given to protect the organisation from potential liabilities, but obviously it causes problems for the university because it doesn't offer a comprehensive summary of your abilities. In these cases the admissions tutor may request an alternative referee from you. This is sometimes done after the interview has taken place and can be a condition of being accepted onto the course.

If you feel that your job will be affected should your employer become aware of your intention to leave, discuss this with the admissions tutor. To protect your employment, the tutor may delay the request for a reference or consider other referees.

Your care colleague

A reference supporting your care experience is going to add strength to your application. This is an ideal opportunity to have someone explain to the admissions team that you have been observed in the care environment and display all the necessary caring characteristics.

You may have several experiences of care, often in different organisations or with different healthcare professionals. Think about these experiences and decide which one gave you the better opportunity to show off your skills.

When requesting a care reference the university asks for information about your:

- ✔ Ability to maintain privacy and dignity
- ✔ Ability to work in a team setting
- ✔ Communication skills
- ✔ Demonstration of compassion
- ✔ General behaviour and attitude
- ✔ Sensitive approach to other people's situations
- ✔ Understanding of confidentially

Your family, friends and acquaintances

As a general rule, references aren't accepted from members of your family, any of your friends or anyone who knows you on a personal basis. The obvious reason for this relates to bias. You can't reasonably expect your mum, dad or best friend to give an objective account of your strengths and weaknesses. They'll only say nice things about you!

For some reason a few candidates don't understand or ignore this rule and use family friends as referees. If you include someone with whom you have a personal relationship as a referee, the admissions tutor will dismiss the reference outright and, because of the competition for places, this dismissal may lead to the rejection of your application.

If you are self-employed or work for the family business then it may be difficult to identify an impartial referee. Contact the university; the admissions tutor will be happy to discuss an alternative person to act as referee.

As long as they don't have a familial relationship to you, the following are normally good referees:

- ✔ A spiritual leader, if you attend a religious group.
- ✔ The organiser of a youth club you attend.
- ✔ The leader of community group you are part of.
- ✔ A professional person, such as a police officer, nurse or justice of the peace.

Looking at the Content of a Reference

References need to give an objective view of your suitability for the role of student nurse. When requesting a reference, the university will explain the role that you have applied for and it may even give some background information on the qualities and attributes which the referee should comment on.

References often contain information relating to your work ethics, such as:

✔ Can you accept constructive criticism, or do you struggle with being told how well you're performing?

✔ Are you industrious and do you complete allocated work, or do you need constant supervision and motivation?

✔ Do you work well as part of a team, or do you have little awareness of team responsibilities?

✔ Are you punctual, or do you struggle with time-keeping?

✔ Can you be trusted, or are you unreliable?

Questions about health or absences aren't normally asked in references but are reviewed once an offer has been made. Absences can be a cause of concern for admissions tutors due to the time limits and professional elements of the programme.

The other element of a reference for student nurses focuses on caring and directs your referee to consider the following:

✔ Are you always polite to others, or can you be rude or abrupt on occasions?

✔ Can you be sensitive to other people's opinions, or do you show little understanding or tolerance for other people's views?

✔ Do you give time to others and show interest in them, or do you display an air of indifference?

✔ Have you a caring disposition, or do you show disregard for others?

✔ Are you considerate of other people's privacy and dignity, or are you lacking an understanding of boundaries?

✔ Do you have good listening skills, or do you show little appreciation of what is being said?

Taking Responsibility for the References

UCAS give you instructions on how to complete your application form and include references. Make sure you follow instructions, as they are slightly different depending on whether you are a school/college student or independent applicant.

References are your responsibility, and you should not expect anyone else to take control of this important feature of your application. Follow the guidance in the following sections to manage your references.

After the reference has been received by the university, they are not obliged to show it or discuss it with you in any detail. You'd have to make a formal application to view the reference and this is both costly and time-consuming. It's much better to know what's expected of your reference than to have any unpleasant shocks.

Keeping an eye on deadlines

Your referee attaches his reference to your online applications. Universities require your references before confirming offers and they often set deadline dates by which the information must be received. Failure to follow directions can result in a rejection of your application.

If your university requires only one reference, you can include it on your application form. An application without a reference looks incomplete and fairs poorly against the competition.

Your application can be delayed in arriving with the admissions tutors if there is a delay in attaching the reference to the UCAS form. Keep in touch with your referee and prompt him to attach his reference to your application.

Should your university require more than one reference, they expect you to provide the necessary details so they can send the request directly to your referee. You're responsible for providing this information and making sure your referee returns the reference to the university on time.

Your application is incomplete without the necessary references. Don't expect the university to follow up and chase any outstanding references. If they have made a request and the information is not returned in a timely fashion, they can reject your application.

Discussing references with referees

Asking permission of someone you want to be your referee is common courtesy. Even if you're still a student and your tutor expects to write a reference for you, it's still polite to ask. Giving people the opportunity to agree to support you also helps them prepare what they'll write.

Chat with the referee about the content of the reference (it's not common practice to actually read the reference yourself). Don't assume that because you liked your boss or worked hard at your job that this means you'll get a glowing reference. Many universities ask for specific information and your referee is obliged to give only the facts; these may not all be to your liking.

Make sure your referee knows which field of nursing you've applied for. It doesn't look good if your reference states you'd make a great adult nurse if you've applied for children's nursing or mental health. Discuss with your referee what the reference is for and the emphasis that is needed, and give him helpful nudges as to your strengths. For more on what kinds of areas the reference covers, see the section 'Looking at the Content of a Reference', earlier in this chapter.

After the reference, stay in touch. You've taken the trouble to ask for a reference and the referee has given his time and effort to write the reference for you. Let him know which universities you have applied to and how your application is progressing. If you succeed, he will be pleased to hear about it. If your application doesn't go to plan, he's more likely to help you prepare a new reference for a future re-application when you've kept him in the loop.

Part V
Attending Selection Days . . . And Beyond

Top Five People You'll Meet at the Selection Day

- **Admissions tutors:** The admissions tutors set the entry criteria for nursing, read and assess your application form and develop the strategies on how you're interviewed. Admissions tutors are a good source of information on everything about your application and how you're taught on the nursing programme.

- **Lecturers:** The largest part of the team on the day is the nurse lecturers. These are the people who, when you start on the programme, teach you while on campus, support your academic study and mark your assignments.

- **Clinical nurses:** As part of your studies you attend clinical practice for half the time. Here you're supported by mentors, registered nurses whose role is to teach you clinical skills, work alongside you while delivering nursing care and assess your clinical competencies.

- **Service users:** Many universities now invite patients and their carers to be involved in selecting students. Service users have experience of what it's like to be cared for, and they understand what characteristics make a good nurse. Be prepared to meet, talk to and get involved with people who have obvious care needs, or even have their carers with them.

- **Students:** The people who know all about being a student, how to survive on the programme and what it takes to succeed are students themselves. It's becoming more popular now for students to have an active role in the selection days, so you could do group work or be asked interview questions by experienced nursing students.

Go to www.dummies.com/extras/getintonursing schooluk for free online bonus content created especially for this book.

In this part . . .

✔ Meet the team who'll assess you on selection days.

✔ Brush up on your numeracy and literacy skills for the tests.

✔ Excel at your interview – and learn interview etiquette.

✔ Assess your options when you're offered a place at nursing school.

✔ Know what to do if you want to defer your place, change your mind or reapply.

Chapter 14

Attending the Selection Day

*T*he accumulation of all your hard work is attending the *selection day* – a day in which, depending on the university's approach, you attend an interview and sit assessments.

Being invited to the selection day means that the admissions tutor has read your reference and reviewed your personal statement. She may even have remembered you from the open day, and she possibly has notes about emails and telephone conversations with you. All this information has led the tutor to believe you have the potential to make a good student. What she now wants to do is meet you in person and see whether you live up to her expectations.

The selection day is your chance to shine – do so, and you'll secure a place; give a lacklustre performance and you may be rejected. This is a highly competitive occasion, so the more background information you have, the better equipped you are to perform well . . . and that's where this chapter comes in.

In this chapter, I explain what to expect on the selection day, from who you'll meet and what you'll do through to considerations like travel arrangements and documents to bring. Reading this chapter alongside Chapter 15 on assessments and Chapter 16 on interviews, you equip yourself to sail through the selection day with flying colours.

Understanding the Basics of Selection Days

Selection days are major events, and it is quite possible for your university to interview hundreds of students in a single day. The admissions team oversee the day, and administrative staff coordinate and manage many of the perfunctory elements.

Your selection day is going to be a busy affair with a lot of hustle and bustle and some waiting around. Having an understanding of the organisation of your event helps you feel a little more relaxed and a lot more prepared.

Running through a typical day

A typical selection day includes the following activities:

- **Signing the register:** On your invite letter you're told where to report on the day. It's important that you follow this instruction so the team know you've arrived. If you don't register your attendance, the team will assume you haven't arrived and you may lose your place.

- **Checking documentation:** If you've been asked to bring documentation with you then at some point the admissions team reviews these. You may be required to hand in your documents for photocopying and to collect them later in the day. These documents are to verify your eligibility for the funding and that you meet entry criteria such as qualifications and the Criminal Records Bureau check.

- **Assessments:** Depending on the type and number of assessments, you may spend a lot of time moving around the campus. Tests such as numeracy and literacy can be conducted on a large scale with many candidates in a single room, but group tasks are usually in teams of five to six candidates. This may require you being divided up and moved into separate rooms, and you get a schedule of where to go and when. Also expect to wear identity badges. Head to Chapter 15 for a detailed look at assessments.

- **Interviews:** There is an interview schedule, and the timing of your interview is pre-arranged. Interviews are normally organised so that those who have the farthest to travel home go first. Expect some waiting around if you're towards the end of the list. Check out Chapter 16 for an in-depth look at the interview.

Identifying the selection team

Each university has its own way of conducting its selection days and uses a team of people who have a vested interest about who should be given a nursing place. These people have undertaken training in selection principles, anti-discriminatory behaviour and equal opportunities and have considerable knowledge about student nurses. The Nursing and Midwifery Council (NMC) makes recommendations on who should be included in the selection process, so expect a variety of people with different experiences to be involved:

- **Admissions tutors:** Admissions tutors are academics who have a specific role to manage the selection of students. They are experienced in selection procedures and have a thorough understanding of good practice when conducting interviews. It is the admissions tutors who set the entry criteria for nursing, read and assess your application form and develop the strategies on how you're interviewed. Due to their expertise in the admissions process, they act as an advisory service for everyone else involved in your interview. With the high number of candidates invited to the selection events, the admissions tutor may not get involved with the actual interviews but oversee the event.

  It's normal for the admissions tutor to have a nursing background with knowledge of your chosen field and the programme of study that you undertake. Admissions tutors are a good source of information on everything about your application and how you are taught on the nursing programme.

- **Lecturers:** The largest part of the team on the day is the nurse lecturers. These are the people who, when you start on the programme, teach you while on campus, support your academic study and mark your assignments. They also act as personal tutors, and so they have insight into the day-to-day issues that students encounter.

  They are all qualified nurses, understand the nursing programme and know what it is like to be a student nurse. They are able to answer many of your questions about the nursing programme and working in clinical practice, plus any of your queries around being a student.

- **Clinical nurses:** As part of your studies you attend clinical practice for half the time. Here you're supported by *mentors*, registered nurses whose role is to teach you clinical skills, work alongside you while delivering nursing care and assess your clinical competencies. These mentors are invited to be involved with your interview, working alongside the lecturers to assess your suitability. Expect to be asked questions from these nurses in relation to your understanding of nursing and clinical practice.

✔ **Service users:** Don't be surprised if you come across people who tell you they have been patients or carers. Nursing has the greatest impact on those who are being cared for, and it is only right that these individuals have a say in choosing who are their future nurses.

Many universities now invite patients and their carers to be involved in selecting students and their opinions are considered alongside everyone else's. Service users have experience of what it's like to be cared for, and they understand what characteristics make a good nurse and those that make a bad nurse. Be prepared to meet, talk to and get involved with people who have obvious care needs, or even have their carers with them.

✔ **Students:** Students are now getting involved with choosing students! The people who know all about being a student, how to survive on the programme and what it takes to succeed are students themselves. It's becoming more popular now for students to have an active role in the selection days, so you could do group work or be asked interview questions by experienced students who are performing well on the programme and have been identified as upholding the professional image of nursing. They give you a good indication of the behaviours you should emulate.

Attending open days is always a good idea so that before the selection day you've familiarised yourself with the campus environment and met some of the admissions team and nursing students.

Scoring candidates

Each university interviews hundreds of students over several selection days. This can make it very difficult to remember who was who and how well every candidate acted without some system of recording their performance.

To make the selection process fair and to categorise candidates against their performance, each university follows guidelines on good practice. Each method of assessment has some structure to it so that you can feel secure in knowing the tasks you are asked to perform. For example, the maths equation you have to work out or the question you are posed is very similar to those every other candidate faces. All the tasks and questions have been pre-planned before the day, and all the interviewing team have been given instructions to ensure consistency.

This structure allows an objective opinion on your suitability to be made, and each task has a marking criteria to allow the admissions team to grade your answer against the task:

✔ Numeracy tests are graded numerically, scoring points for each correct answer. Some tests may use negative marking which deducts a point for incorrect answers.

✔ Written tests are scored numerically or as a percentage. Scores are given for content, comprehension, grammar and spelling.

✔ Group work tasks normally examine teamwork, communication and problem-solving skills. Scores are either numerical or by expressive grade such as *excellent*, *satisfactory* and *poor*.

✔ Interviews can have many themes, from understanding care and demonstration of commitment to appreciation of current issues. Scoring is usually through numerical or expressive grading.

Universities tell you what the pass mark is for the numeracy and literacy tests and will explain if they allow for a resit. You may not be told the pass score for the group-work tasks or face-to-face interview before the actual event, as this may be determined by the calibre of candidates who attend and the score may change from year to year.

The overall decision on whether to offer a place or not is made by considering how well the applicant did during the face-to-face interview, what percentage was awarded for numeracy and the grade awarded for literacy.

Getting Ready for Selection Days

Preparation is the key ingredient to a calm and stress-free selection day. Well, maybe not quite stress free, but why increase the stress by being disorganised! A little knowledge and planning goes a long way to making sure everything runs as smoothly as possible for you.

Confirming your attendance

The first you hear about a selection day is in an invite letter, in which a university invites you to attend.

The selection days are chosen to coincide with the UCAS application cycle, and several dates are arranged to ensure that all the interviews and assessments are concluded and decisions made by the required UCAS dates. You can find the timeline for the university to make decisions on the UCAS website (www.ucas.com), but generally if you have applied before 15 January, the university makes a decision by the beginning of April.

Some universities offer you a selection of dates, which is good because you can self-select the most appropriate date for you. Other universities, however, don't give this option and offer one date only.

Consider the date carefully:

✔ Does it coincide with school or college work, and can you miss these lessons?

✔ When are your exams? Does the interview disrupt them?

✔ Will the date conflict with other universities' dates you may be attending?

If the date really isn't ideal for you, look into your options for requesting a change in date. It's at the discretion of the university whether they change your interview date. Universities are accommodating, but with such large numbers of candidates and few interview dates, they may not offer you an alternative date.

 Always confirm that you're attending the interview. If the university asks you to confirm and you don't, they can offer your place to another candidate and turn you away. Don't expect them to squeeze you in!

Collecting documents and paperwork

The amount of paperwork required is astounding, but remember that the university must make numerous checks to ensure your eligibility to start the course. As a brief reminder, original paperwork is needed for:

✔ Checking your eligibility for the course fees.

✔ Identifying the level of bursary you will receive.

✔ Knowing your tax and loan entitlements.

✔ Making sure you have the right academic qualifications.

✔ Reviewing your good character status.

✔ Assessing your physical health and wellbeing.

The university asks for at least some of this information on the selection day. It may be the case that only a selection of the documents is required at this time, and the other documents could be requested at various other points in the selection process. However, because you need to produce all these documents at some point, have everything prepared by the selection day stage. Have these documents photocopied and ready to provide to the university alongside the originals.

The amount of documentation that you need depends on your personal circumstances, but as a rule have the following available:

- ✔ Academic certificates
- ✔ The written report about the help you require if you have a learning need such as dyslexia
- ✔ Birth certificate
- ✔ Birth certificates of any children whom you wish to claim financial support for
- ✔ Change of name deed
- ✔ Driving licence
- ✔ Evidence of any tax allowances
- ✔ Evidence of right to remain in the UK
- ✔ Marriage certificate
- ✔ Passport
- ✔ Utility bill

Some universities cancel the interview if you don't bring along the required documents. Double-check you have all that's requested, and place all of your documents in your bag the night before. I've lost count of the number of candidates who left them on the kitchen table! And remember to collect all your documents before returning home.

Planning your outfit

First impressions count for a lot. You don't have much time to impress the admissions team, and the way you dress can help demonstrate your motivation. Two approaches exist:

- ✔ **The knowledgeable candidate:** Some admissions tutors don't consider dress code as too much of an issue. Within the bounds of reasonableness, the interviewers are happy for you to express yourself through the clothes you wear. These tutors concentrate on what you have to say and think about nursing and the profession.

✔ **The professional candidate:** Although all admissions tutors agree that candidates must demonstrate knowledge of nursing, some also consider the level of professionalism that you display. Making an effort at interview and attending smartly dressed can show that you understand the importance of displaying a professional image.

Whichever approach you agree with, consider the following:

✔ Think about what your competition will be wearing. Will your dress sense put you at a disadvantage?

✔ You have to travel and sit in the same clothes for quite a few hours, so choose clothes that are comfortable to wear.

✔ Keeping warm or staying cool is important. You don't want to be distracted by an uncomfortable temperature.

✔ New and expensive clothes aren't required; what is essential are clean and neatly pressed clothes. The dishevelled look is not going to impress!

✔ Be sensitive to others. Are any of the logos or pictures on your clothes, your tattoos or piercings upsetting or offensive?

Making travel arrangements

One of the frequent disturbances to the smooth running of selection days is the interruptions made by candidates arriving late. The admissions team plan their events to take into account the travelling of candidates, and they accommodate some lateness; however, should you arrive too late, you may well miss your interview and/or assessment. Don't expect the admissions team to delay the interviews and assessments because you haven't arrived on time; other candidates who did arrive on time shouldn't be kept waiting.

To avoid tardiness:

✔ Check the time, date and venue of your appointment.

✔ If possible, do a practice run of travelling to the campus.

✔ Use route planners to estimate your journey time.

✔ Take into account rush hour traffic and road works.

✔ If travelling by train, give yourself time for all the connections.

✔ Know where to park or where to catch a taxi or bus.

✔ Travel the night before if you'll struggle to do the journey in the morning.

Also note the time the session finishes. You don't want to book your return journey too early and have to leave the session before it ends. Give yourself plenty of breathing space.

If, on the day, you have a disaster and fall behind, make sure you call the admissions tutor immediately and explain the situation. And don't be afraid to ask for directions if you're lost!

Keeping contact details current

Double-check that your contact details are updated on your UCAS form; the university may need to contact you. Also make sure you have to hand all the contact details you need for the university, including the telephone number of the person who sent you the invite letter. Once you have started your journey you need to be able to keep in touch.

Coping on the Day

How you manage the selection day is important as it's likely to be the only occasion where you can make a personal impact on the admissions team. The day can be stressful, especially if you have no experience of selection days or interviews, but in this section I give you a few tips to prepare yourself and control those stressors that impact on your performance.

Weighing up the competition

It may be strange thinking along the lines of who else is invited to the selection days, but these are your competitors, and so it is well worth giving them some consideration. The university hopes to select the best students and draws its candidates based on potential more than any other criteria. The staff must comply with the Equality Act, so don't be surprised if the admissions team spend more time with some candidates or make slight alterations to the planning of the day; it's to ensure all are treated fairly.

You'll meet candidates:

- ✔ Of varying ages; I've interviewed candidates in their teens, 20s, 30s, 40s and 50s.
- ✔ From both genders, though more women apply than men.
- ✔ From different ethnic and cultural backgrounds.
- ✔ Who have travelled long distances to attend.

✔ Who need adjustments for health or learning reasons.

✔ With a variety of care experience.

Some of the candidates attending with you may also be success-ful and could be a member of your cohort. Friendships can start even at this stage of nursing! You may want to take a few emails or telephone numbers to maintain contact with other applicants from your selection event.

During the course of the day you'll no doubt be left sitting with other candidates for some periods while you wait. Those candidates are feeling just the same as you. Yes, they are your competitors, but they're also your future classmates, so treat them as such. Chatting together can help alleviate anxiety, and for many candidates this won't be their first interview, so you can share hints and tips. Remember that lasting friendships can start at this encounter.

Although the admissions team are busy during these events, they do observe your conduct throughout the day. Your attitude and behaviour towards other candidates is noted and can be used to gain an overall impression of your suitability for nursing.

Controlling the signals you send out

The admissions team fully expects you to be anxious about your interview and quite nervous. It is not their intention to make you feel this way, and they do attempt to put you at ease. They under-stand that to get the best from you they need to make you relaxed and comfortable.

However, regardless of how you feel, you have to perform well and impress the team. They are observing your behaviour and your responses to the assessments and interview questions, so you need to ensure that *all* the signals you give out are positive ones. The following sections help you consider the verbal and non-ver-bal signals you give.

Dealing with family and friends

Many candidates bring along family members or friends for support. This is quite acceptable and helps calm your nerves. But keep in mind that people you bring with you aren't allowed to get involved with assessments, and there are no child-care facilities, so they'll have to head off to other university facilities or local attractions. And at the end of the day you'll need to find each other again – the admissions team may have a plan for this, or give instructions for where and when to meet.

Verbal signals

The NMC requires all students to have 'good command of spoken English'. So you must demonstrate the ability to use English in formal and informal conversations.

You get many opportunities during the selection day to demonstrate your oral skills and for the team to gain an impression of how well you can communicate. Verbal communication is consciously assessed in the tasks and interviews, but also by observing you throughout the day.

Follow these pointers to impress the selection team:

✔ Use appropriate language that shows you have command of how you speak. Slang and swear words such as 'brill' instead of 'brilliant' or 'cock-up' instead of 'mistake' don't give a good impression!

✔ Be sensitive to others who are listening to you, as you don't want to upset other candidates by off-the-cuff remarks or jokes about their performance, dress sense or abilities.

✔ Practise what you want to say. Hearing the words out loud is very different to saying them in your head.

✔ Have someone to listen to you. What sounds good to you may not sound so good to others, and although you know what you're trying to say it may not be so clear to someone else.

✔ Consider your accent. You'll be with candidates from different regions of the country and dialects differ. Don't assume all candidates speak like you, so be sure you're making yourself clear.

✔ Consider the tone and pace of your speech during the interview. Having a calm tone and talking at a normal speed shows you to be more in control of the situation, whereas excited and rushed talking or slow and confused speech gives a poor impression.

✔ Engage in conversation and put expression in your voice to show interest.

For more pointers on interview preparation, go to Chapter 16.

Non-verbal signals

Throughout the interview day you must demonstrate the right attitude and behaviour expected of nursing candidates (for more on nursing attributes, head to Chapter 5). You are judged on the way you portray yourself in your interactions and engagement with others. This means that at all times you should be thinking how to present yourself well.

Here are some tips to help you stand out for the right reasons:

✓ Take every opportunity to be involved with others. You want to give an impression of being able to relate to others.

✓ Use your body language to show interest, maintain eye contact and use facial expressions to engage with others. Place yourself close enough to other candidates so they can talk with you easily, and keep your arms unfolded and legs uncrossed. These all give a positive impression.

✓ If clinical suites or books and articles have been made available for you on the day, use them to show interest.

✓ If you need to scream, do so quietly in the washrooms!

Heading home at the end of the day

After all the excitement and charged energy of preparing yourself for the day, and then sitting the assessments and/or having an interview, the ending of the event can be an anticlimax. With some selection days you have no gathering at the end to review how the day went, and candidates are left to leave the campus on their own and go their separate ways. You can leave quite drained and exhausted and also a little downbeat. This is to be expected, so plan the rest of the day to get yourself through these feelings:

✓ Arrange a pickup point if meeting with family and friends so you're not waiting around.

✓ Have someone to drive, because your mind is on other things.

✓ Treat yourself to something special to help you relax, such as a meal or drink with friends.

✓ Don't fret and attempt to analyse what you did right or wrong; you've time to recap on the event another day.

Chapter 15

Preparing for Assessments

. . . .

In This Chapter

▶ Finding out whether you'll attend assessments

▶ Looking at different types of assessment

▶ Knowing what to expect and how to prepare

. . . .

*Y*our academic qualifications and personal achievements written in your application form are a good starting point to demonstrate your abilities. However, the information in the form doesn't always translate into usable skills in the clinical environment, and in some cases academically capable students are unable to safely practise nursing roles. So many universities require additional proof of your skills and abilities demonstrated during assessments.

In this chapter, I explain the different assessments you have to sit: numeracy, literacy and group work. By the end of this chapter you'll have a good idea of what to expect on assessment day and how you can prepare.

As with any assessments, your performance is monitored and scored. At the end of the selection event the admissions tutor adds all of your scores and grades together to give a picture of your ability and potential; gaining the best total possible improves your chances of receiving an offer of a place.

 Performing well with the tests and assessments shows that you have the underpinning knowledge and attitude needed to start the nursing programme. This gives confidence to the admissions team that with the right support and teaching you have the potential to develop into a good nursing student.

 If you have a diagnosis of a learning need and have a specific action plan of support then contact the university in advance of the assessment date. They'll be happy to arrange support if given enough warning to make preparations.

Finding Out About Tests

There is no straightforward way of knowing whether your chosen university tests or not, so a little detective work is needed:

- ✔ Check the university information on UCAS. Often information about the type of assessment at interview is given in the 'Course Specific Requirements' section.

- ✔ Read through the university website. Often information is available to explain the selection assessments, and many websites give example numeracy or literacy tests so you can familiarise yourself before the event.

So, you should know pre-application whether you'll need to sit tests. When you receive your letter inviting you to interview you'll find information and sometimes samples included.

Universities don't have to test candidates, so the practice of assessing and how assessments are conducted varies across the UK. You may find that from your choices you only need to attend an interview for one university, whereas another expects you to be interviewed and sit a numeracy and literacy test.

As with the variation in testing, there is also a variation in how the tests are conducted and how you receive your results. Some universities incorporate the tests into interview days, but others keep them separate. Here are a few examples you may encounter:

- ✔ Sit the tests and have the interview the same the day. The decision is made through UCAS as an offer or unsuccessful.

- ✔ Sit the tests in the morning. If you pass the tests you have your interview in the afternoon.

- ✔ You attend on one day for the tests and are informed whether you passed or not. If successful, you attend a second date for your interview.

Tests take place at the university, but the location may be different to that of your interview or to where nursing is taught. Make sure you read the instructions carefully before planning your travel arrangements. Turning up at the wrong place and missing your assessment can lead to rejection.

When inviting you to attend a selection event, universities give you information on what to expect on the day. Most provide examples of assessments to help you prepare, either on their website or included with your invite letter.

Exploring Numeracy Tests

Nurses require a range of numeracy skills to perform their daily roles. Drug calculations are the main priority, but in a typical working day you can be expected to use your numeracy skills in many tasks, such as:

- ✔ Assessing monitor information
- ✔ Calculating fluid balance
- ✔ Checking body temperature
- ✔ Completing time sheets
- ✔ Filling out charts
- ✔ Managing money
- ✔ Measuring blood pressure

Your university has numeracy assessments built into the nursing programme and you're tested when on campus as well as in clinical practice. It is very likely that by the end of the programme you must achieve 100 per cent in your numeracy tests, so the admissions tutors need to assess that you have basic numeracy skills.

What to expect

Each university that assesses numeracy does so differently, but all assess fundamental numeracy skills. You need to be able to understand and calculate numbers, such as:

- ✔ Percentages and fractions
- ✔ Ratios
- ✔ Weights and volumes

Here's a selection of typical questions that cover the fundamental numeracy skills. Note that some are stated as pure mathematical examples and others are described in a problem-solving format based in social and nursing situations.

1. What is $125 - 28$?

2. Calculate $23.08 - 12.1$.

3. What is 12.5% of 200?

4. Reduce this fraction to its lowest term: $^{290}\!/_{580}$.

5. How many millilitres in $\frac{3}{5}$ of a litre?

6. Round this number up to one decimal place: 63.47.

7. A sweet shop sells the following: fizzy bombs – 13; sugar snaps – 24; sour drops – 19; candy flops – 7. How many sweets were sold all together?

8. A nurse takes the blood pressure of 60 patients. Thirty per cent of the recordings were high. How many patients had high blood pressure?

9. An ambulance travels at an average speed of 32 kph. It travels a distance of 56 km from the patient's home to hospital. How long does the journey take?

10. A tank for home heating contains 288 litres of oil. It takes 18 litres of oil to heat the home each day. How many days can the tank heat the home?

11. A patient's temperature rises from 37.2 to 38.7°C. By now much does the temperature increase?

12. Five hundred patients visit the clinic during the week. The ratio of female to male patients is 3:1. How many male patients visit the clinic?

Answers: 1. 97; 2. 10. 98; 3. 25; 4. 1 /2; 5. 400; 6. 63.5; 7. 63; 8. 18; 9. 1 hour 45; 10. 16; 11. 1.5; 12. 125.

Each university has its own pass mark for numeracy tests – usually, approximately 50 per cent, although some can be higher.

How to prepare

You're given instructions for preparation with your invite letter, but also think about the following tips as you prepare:

✔ If a calculator is allowed, make sure you're familiar with how one works. You can't use your mobile phone to make calculations.

✔ The assessment is time constrained between 20 and 40 minutes. Try answering your revision questions against the clock.

✔ You could have to answer 10 to 20 questions, so plan 1 to 2 minutes each.

✔ Show your workings out, so you can develop the logic of your answers in your revision.

Some hospitals have put together helpful hints for numeracy test preparation. Visit www.snap.nhs.uk for more information.

Getting to Grips with Literacy Tests

In the context of the nursing course assessment, literacy is about having good skills in reading, writing and comprehension of language. Having good literacy skills is essential in nursing. You need to understand and interpret what you read and also write clearly, accurately and meaningfully.

As a student nurse you're expected to use your literacy skills to:

✔ Complete charts and forms with legible and precise information.

✔ Read books and articles and understand their meaning.

✔ Review clinical documents and case notes and gain an accurate impression of the issues.

✔ Write accounts of your clinical care that others can understand.

✔ Write essays that demonstrate your level of knowledge.

To understand the importance of literacy in clinical practice, read the Nursing and Midwifery Council's guidance on record keeping, which you can find on its website: www.nmc-uk.org.

What to expect

Literacy skills can be assessed in various ways, but the popular methods of testing include undertaking a handwriting task, a test of your reading skills and a spelling test. Tests commonly assess:

✔ Comprehension

✔ Grammar

✔ Punctuation

✔ Spelling

The admissions tutors concentrate on the basic reading and writing skills, and expect you to have the ability to write clearly and legibly. Here are five example questions to give you an idea of how universities present literacy tests:

1. Read the following text:

   The core temperature of the human body remains almost constant, and although there is no 'normal' temperature, the average is generally considered to be between 36–37.6°C. In contrast, skin temperature will fluctuate according to the temperature of the surrounding environment. Body temperature is important for homeostasis, as cells are temperature-sensitive and can function only within a narrow temperature range.

As environmental temperatures are too low for normal cell function to occur, the body produces its own heat as a by-product of metabolism. The energy produced through metabolism is measured by calculating the basal metabolic rate (BMR), which is the minimum amount of energy required to maintain the functions of the body when at rest. The minimum BMR can account for 60% of daily energy expenditure. Heat is also produced as a result of muscle activity, digestion and hormone activity. Not all the energy produced is used by the body and any excess of free energy is lost as heat.

(From Evered, A. (2003) Hypothermia: risk factors and guidelines for nursing care. *Nursing Times*; 99:49, 40–43.)

Write a short summary in your own words of between 4 to 6 lines to show what you understand about the passage.

2. 'The boy . . . upset when his toy broke.' Which word or phrase correctly completes the sentence?

    a. will become

    b. went

    c. is

    d. became

3. Which word is spelt correctly?

    a. Stethascope

    b. Stephascope

    c. Stethoscope

    d. Stephoscope

4. When washing their hands, nurses must <u>strictly follow</u> hospital policies. Which words have the same meaning as those underlined?

    a. Seriously consider

    b. Abide by

    c. Agree with

    d. Think about

5. You have 20 minutes to write an essay on ONE of the following topics. Your essay should be approximately 500 words.

   a. Discuss why you have chosen your particular field of nursing.

   b. Describe the qualities of a good nurse.

Answers: 2. d; 3. c.; 4. b.

How to prepare

Brush up on your spelling, grammar and punctuation (*English Grammar For Dummies* can help!). Ensure you break up long paragraphs when writing. In comprehension exercises, if you struggle at first to understand a passage, read it out loud to yourself or write comments alongside the text as each part starts to make sense to you.

The BBC has a comprehensive revision site that many universities recommend using to help you prepare for your numeracy and literacy assessments. Visit www.bbc.co.uk/skillswise.

Doing Practical Assessments

Practical assessments move away from testing academic qualities and focus upon the emotional and behavioural aspects of nursing. Many universities use practical activities to gain insight into your attitude towards caring and also towards other people. These activities usually assess:

✔ Ability to work within a group setting.

✔ Attitude towards care.

✔ Behaviour around other people.

✔ Problem-solving skills.

✔ Your understanding of healthcare.

What to expect

Practical activities can be arranged in several ways depending on the system used. The practical work usually has more structure, and you can expect to:

✔ Be on your own or in a group of 3 to 6 candidates.

✔ Move between work stations or classrooms.

> ✔ Have a series of tasks to perform or problems to solve (usually, each lasts around 20 minutes).
>
> ✔ Take various roles during the tasks.

Here are some types of tasks and an example of each:

> ✔ **The lone task:** You have to explain to a patient (played by an actor) that they can't go home from hospital as the ambulance wasn't booked in time. The patient may be given prior instructions to become very upset.
>
> You're observed dealing with the situation and need to consider:
>
> • Your verbal response.
>
> • Your non-verbal signals.
>
> • How to make a connection with the patient.
>
> ✔ **The health-related task:** Your group must consider a health-related topic that's currently in the media. You have to agree on the topic and discuss its implications. You are expected to present the findings of your discussions as a means of a debate. You:
>
> • Define the topic and explain the media reports.
>
> • Give a discussion on pros of the topic.
>
> • Debate the cons of the topic.
>
> • Offer a final discussion on the group's standpoint.
>
> ✔ **The task to assess teamwork, communication and problem-solving skills (may not be healthcare related):** Your group has to construct a bridge that's capable of supporting a stapler. You have four plastic cups and plates, several sheets of paper and a roll of tape.

How to prepare

These assessments are concerned with your attitudes and behaviours as well as your problem-solving and communication skills. Your attitudes are part of who you are, which may make it difficult to change. However, it is possible to change your behaviours before attending the assessments, and you can revise your problem-solving and communication skills.

Here are some good ways to prepare:

> ✔ Use any care experience you have to reflect on how patients and carers work together.

✔ Listen to the news and read newspapers to find out what the media think makes a good nurse (or a not-so-good one).

✔ People watch. Observe how people interact with each other and look for the cues of good interpersonal skills.

✔ Look back on times when you had to find the solution to a problem and think about the stages you went through to achieve your goal.

Chapter 16

Excelling in the Interview

● ●

In This Chapter

▶ Exploring the interview process

▶ Perfecting etiquette

▶ Gaining interview practice

▶ Preparing for questions

▶ Planning your own questions

● ●

*W*hen selecting future students, each university is required to follow the guidelines of the Nursing and Midwifery Council (NMC), which include the admissions tutor having 'face-to-face engagement' with you before making a decision. Remember that a significant part of your education is in clinical practice, working with and caring for vulnerable and ill people. The university has a responsibility to ensure you have the right attitude and behaviour to be part of the nursing team.

The most popular way to assess your suitability for nursing is to use the classic interview approach in which you're in the spotlight and answer a number of questions posed by either an interviewer or a small team of interviewers (for the lowdown on who interviews you, head to Chapter 14).

Interviews can be very stressful occasions. Many candidates find it difficult to express themselves in the way they'd like and often feel they could have performed much better. In the short time you have to 'blow your own trumpet', you can waste opportunities through fear and worry of the interview process itself, rather than concentrating on how to show yourself in the best light possible.

Don't worry – in this chapter, I eliminate your interview discomfort by explaining exactly what the interview process entails so you know what to expect. Then I give you the lowdown on interview practice, and offer plenty of examples of types of questions you'll be asked, so that you can walk into the interview room feeling ready and confident.

Following the Three Stages of the Interview

In the face-to-face interview, regardless of how it's organised, your interview proceeds through stages. The order and timing of the phases differ slightly between universities, but expect your interview to go through these three stages.

Warming up

The warm-up stage is the most important, even though it accounts for only a small amount of the time you spend in the interview. In this stage the interviewer aims to:

✔ Settle you into the interview

✔ Build an initial rapport with you

✔ Explain how the interview will proceed

The interviewer will be polite, courteous and friendly; she understands your feelings of stress and anxiety. Her intention is to put you at ease as much as possible so you feel confident in answering her questions. She asks easy-to-answer 'ice-breaking' questions that help you settle into the interview, such as:

✔ **'Tell me a little about yourself. . . .'** Don't tell the interviewer your life history, say a little about your family, your hobbies or interests. Don't start saying why you want to be a nurse at this point.

✔ **'How far have you travelled today and how was your journey?'** Don't complain about problems you encountered while travelling to the university, say whether you travelled with family or friends and even mention the weather if you like!

✔ **'Have you been to the university before?'** Don't just say 'yes' or 'no' – elaborate a little. If you've attended the open day or recognise the admissions tutor, say so. Doing so gives a good impression.

It can take as little as four minutes for the interviewer to gain an impression of how well the interview is going and to progress and decide about your suitability for nursing. So how you act and behave in these first few moments is vital in gaining the advantage and ensuring the rest of the interview develops in your favour.

Questions and answers

This is the main stage of the interview. Time-wise, this is the longest part of the interview, during which the interviewer explores your reasons for applying to nursing. The interviewer is looking to:

- ✔ Discuss why you have chosen a particular field of nursing.
- ✔ Explore your commitment to nursing.
- ✔ Identify what motivates you in relation to caring.
- ✔ Review your understanding of the academic side of the nursing programme.
- ✔ Examine individual characteristics mentioned in your personal statement.

The interviewer understands that you may find some questions easier to answer than others, but she expects you to attempt all the questions. To do so:

- ✔ Don't answer immediately. Give yourself a few seconds to understand the question.
- ✔ Be clear what is being asked. If you don't understand the question, ask for it to be rephrased.
- ✔ If you really don't know the answer, say so. The interviewer appreciates your honesty more than you rambling on in an obvious attempt to hide your ignorance.

Listening is just as powerful as talking. Interviewers often give clues to the answers in their questions.

Winding down

Depending on how the university has planned the interview schedule, the winding down stage may include several elements:

- ✔ **Your questions:** You have the opportunity to ask the interviewer questions (see the later section 'Questioning the Selectors').
- ✔ **Portfolio review:** If the opportunity did not arise during the question and answer stage, the interviewer may want to review any documentation that you have brought to support your interview.

✔ **Administrative checks:** Sometimes the interviewer asks questions related to the interview and selection process. These are usually to ensure you have been given all the correct information such as start dates, conditions of any offers and expectations of travelling to clinical practice. You don't need to prepare answers for these questions.

✔ **What happens next:** The interviewer gives you information on the next stage, such as when a decision will be made, whether you need to do anything else after leaving the interview room or how to leave the building now that your interview has ended.

Usually, this stage feels less intensive than the questions and answers one. This is still part of the interview, so don't relax too much and undo all your hard work. Maintain the good impression built up throughout the interview so you leave the interviewer with a positive image of nursing potential.

Getting Smart about Interview Etiquette

Interview etiquette is about behaving in the fashion deemed appropriate for a selection event. Nursing's social code is that of professionalism, caring and compassion (for more on the people side of nursing, check out Chapter 5), so those are qualities you need to project.

Seeing how interviewers prepare

Universities work to codes of practice and do their utmost to make the interview a positive experience for you. A lot of preparation goes on before meeting you:

✔ Arranging the interview teams for each group of candidates.

✔ Planning the timing for each interview.

✔ Deciding on the themes for the questions.

✔ Setting similar questions to be asked of each candidate.

✔ Allowing time for each interviewer to read the candidate's UCAS application.

✔ Ensuring that each candidate is being treated fairly and equally.

Here's how you can demonstrate excellent interview etiquette:

- ✔ Arrive ten minutes early for your interview.

- ✔ Be courteous. Address the interviewer by her full title unless asked to do otherwise, and don't sit until invited to do so.

- ✔ Wear appropriate attire. Wear comfortable clothes that aren't too short or tight. Avoid jeans, especially if they're ripped!

- ✔ Maintain eye contact.

- ✔ Have a positive body posture. Don't sit rigidly. Try to relax, put your bag, coat and paperwork down on a desk or under the chair so you aren't clutching onto your personal possessions. And you don't want the contents of your bag sliding onto the floor!

- ✔ Use good diction and demonstrate control of the English language. Avoid slang and expletives.

- ✔ Be thorough with your answers and concise with your words.

- ✔ Give opinions; avoid bland replies. But make sure your views are fair, not discriminatory or patronising. And never be forceful in your opinions to the point of being argumentative.

- ✔ Be honest if you don't know an answer. Don't make excuses.

- ✔ Show enthusiasm about being a student nurse. Focus on what you can bring to nursing, not what nursing means to you.

- ✔ Be informed: show knowledge about nursing and the nursing programme. You're also demonstrating your ability to study at degree level and so reveal your potential to cope with the course demands as well.

Mirror your interviewer's approach to the interview. If she remains formal in her posture and questioning, do the same. If she's relaxed and allows some informality in the interview then be a little more relaxed yourself.

Getting Experience of Interviews

Very few people have ample interview experience to make them feel confident in the interview setting. If you're like most people then many years go by between job hunting or promotion before you need to think about interview practice. Yet how you perform at interview is often the deciding factor in whether you secure the position applied for.

Practising your interview skills helps relieve stress at the actual interview. Being confident in what you want to say and how you want to say it allows you to concentrate more on engaging with the interviewer rather than worrying about your answers.

Treat the interview in the same way as you have the whole selection process. Plan far ahead in anticipation that at some point you'll have to present yourself in front of a selection team and perform well.

Usually, candidates perform reasonably well but don't shine. Mastering the art of the interview can make the difference between a good interview and an excellent interview.

Your interview experience needs to be realistic and give you the opportunity to:

- ✔ Feel the pressure of answering questions.
- ✔ Understand the tension of unfamiliar surroundings.
- ✔ Conduct yourself in front of a stranger.
- ✔ Hear yourself talking out loud in a structured way.
- ✔ Realise how much you know and don't know about nursing.

You could use many opportunities to gain experience. Your school or college may arrange interview days where they invite organisations in your area of interest to come and offer mock interviews. But also consider asking any of the following to interview you:

- ✔ A work colleague, preferably with some management experience.
- ✔ Your neighbour or family friend who can be constructive in her feedback.
- ✔ A close friend who's honest in identifying your strengths and weaknesses.

To help your mock interviewer act out her role, write out a selection of the questions from this chapter for her to use (see the next section). If the interviewer doesn't have experience of healthcare, she can still ask appropriate questions for you to answer.

Rehearsing Your Answers

The more familiar you are with the type of questions that are likely to be asked at interview, the more you can rehearse answers and so feel confident in your responses on the day.

You can plan your answers in advance, but be ready to adapt or change them to the specific question. You're soon found out if your answers are too scripted.

When rehearsing, talk out loud to get used to hearing your voice, and record yourself speaking to help you identify issues. Watch out for:

✔ Using the same word often – make a list of alternatives to use instead.

✔ Caring terminology – use it to help focus your answers, but avoid other jargon.

✔ Distracting mannerisms – for example, do you say 'you know' a lot?

✔ Facts backing up your opinions – make sure your views have a good grounding.

The following sections help you get to grips with the kinds of questions you'll get, and how to answer them.

Understanding the types of question

The interviewers ask questions in a way that requires a different response based on the information they need to know. Expect a combination of the following types of questions:

✔ **Closed-ended questions:** These are confirmation questions mostly used either at the beginning or the end of the interview. They require only a brief reply or single word response, such as 'yes' or 'no'. These questions are normally used to clarify facts such as qualifications, work experience and contact details.

✔ **Open-ended questions:** These questions make up the middle stage of the interview. They require a lengthy response by you in which you demonstrate your depth of knowledge around the subject. Your answers must tell the interviewer that you understand nursing and healthcare and what it means to be a nursing student.

Open-ended questions divide into three categories:

• Traditional questions

• Behavioural questions

• Situational questions

Traditional questions

These are the questions that you'd expect to be asked at interview. They're often about you and your circumstances or aspirations, such as:

- What triggered your interest in applying to train as a nurse??
- What is your greatest strength?
- Where do you see yourself in five years' time?
- What makes you better than the other candidates?

Behavioural questions

These questions concentrate on your past experiences. The idea is that by demonstrating your previous attitude and behaviour the interviewer can predict how you might perform as a nursing student.

The interviewer asks questions that require you to explain how you acted in real-world situations in which you demonstrated attributes that match those expected of a student nurse.

Here are some examples:

- Give an example of when you showed compassion to someone.
- Demonstrate how you used good communication in your last job.
- Describe an occasion when someone relied on you for help.
- Give an example of when you managed your stress effectively.

Use the STAR system to shape your answer for these questions:

- **Situation:** Briefly describe the background to the event.
- **Task:** Explain the activity that demonstrated your behaviour or attitude.
- **Action:** Describe what steps you took and why in order to use the skill or behaviour.
- **Result:** Outline the outcome of your action as a positive achievement of the skill or behaviour mentioned in the question.

Situational questions

These questions pose hypothetical situations that allow the interviewer to find out how you would approach certain problems.

Unlike behavioural questions that require you to discuss an actual experience you've encountered, these questions consider your responses to a situation should it occur in the future.

Examples include:

✔ How would you react if a patient was verbally aggressive?

✔ What would you do if your patient was in pain?

✔ What issues would you consider when taking a client to the bathroom?

✔ Imagine seeing another healthcare worker being rude to a resident. What would you do?

These types of questions appear quite daunting. However, with some organisation and understanding of what the interviewer wants, they're quite easy to manage. You aren't expected to know everything about nursing, but you are expected to have common sense and a basic understanding of nursing values such as dignity, respect, professionalism, advocacy and so on.

Plan for these types of questions in four steps:

1. Research the role of the nurse and understand the common principles and values that underpin nursing.

2. Read around the various roles for your field of nursing to give you some vision of likely clinical situations.

3. Try to link the principles and values in Step 1 with the clinical situations in Step 2.

4. Read some nursing articles or recent media reports where care has not been as good as expected, and try to think which of the nursing principles and values could be used to make the situation better.

Being aware of the types of questions asked makes it much easier to rehearse your responses, because you understand what's expected from each type of question.

Looking at typical questions

It is difficult to predict precisely which questions the interviewer will ask, all university nursing interviews focus on the same themes. Reviewing your answers against the following examples gives you sufficient knowledge to adapt your answers to alternative questions each university may ask.

When posing questions the interviewer considers not only your answer but also your:

- ✔ Appreciation of current healthcare issues.
- ✔ Commitment to nursing.
- ✔ Communication skills.
- ✔ Motivation to pursue your chosen field.
- ✔ Understanding of the role of the nurse.

The following sections offer examples of questions within the main themes the interviewer explores.

Questions about choice of field

On your UCAS form you indicate which field of nursing you want to work in. The interviewer wants to know why this field interests you and that you have a good understanding of what nursing in this field entails.

Here are some example questions:

- ✔ Tell me why you've chosen adult nursing.
- ✔ Explain what you think learning disability students do in a typical shift.
- ✔ You've chosen adult nursing but your experiences on your personal statement are about mental health. Why is this?
- ✔ What qualities do you think are needed to work with mental health patients?
- ✔ On your application form you have applied to midwifery and children's nursing. Do you think they are similar fields of nursing?

Questions regarding education and learning

The nursing programme isn't all about clinical practice and you do need to meet the academic standards to be awarded the degree. The interviewer needs you to demonstrate a healthy attitude towards study and an appreciation of what a degree in nursing entails.

Example questions include:

- ✔ Explain how you think you will be taught and assessed on the nursing programme.
- ✔ Why do you think it's important that nurses are educated to degree level?

✔ Please give an example of how you've recently revised and studied for your exams.

✔ Can you explain the relationship between clinical practice and academic study on this programme?

✔ What's your greatest challenge in coming to university?

Questions determining understanding of the profession

It may surprise you, but many candidates struggle when asked to talk about nursing. They can use nursing jargon, but can't explain what nurses do in any detail. The interviewers are looking for candidates who appreciate what a career in nursing means.

Be prepared for questions like these:

✔ What is the role of a registered nurse?

✔ What do you think the role of the nurse is in the multidisciplinary healthcare team?

✔ Where do you hope to be in five years' time, and what do you think you have to do to get there?

✔ What do you think is different about nursing that makes it stand out from other healthcare professions?

✔ Give an example of when you have helped someone that could be used to show your nursing qualities.

Questions demonstrating management of commitments

Student nurses have to work harder and for longer than many other university students. One of the biggest challenges to students is managing their many commitments and keeping on track to qualify as a nurse. The interviewer needs to know that you understand the level of commitment necessary to complete the programme.

Prepare for these questions:

✔ Give an example of when you've managed several commitments successfully.

✔ What coping mechanisms do you use to manage your stress?

✔ What action would you take if you were struggling with your workload?

✔ Tell me about a decision that you have made recently that had a positive effect upon managing your time.

✔ What do you think the challenges are for you when working in clinical practice and having academic work to complete?

Questions to illustrate attitude towards care

The interview team expect you to demonstrate a suitable attitude towards care. They want to know that you aren't discriminatory or likely to behave in a way that harms or upsets others. Asking questions relating to care gives insight into your intrinsic values and morals.

Here are some example questions:

✔ You have been asked to wash a patient before breakfast. The patient, however, doesn't want a wash until after breakfast. What will you do?

✔ A resident wants to stay in bed all day, but her plan of care to promote independent living states she should go out shopping. How would you manage the situation?

✔ Please give me an example of how you showed compassion to someone else.

✔ Explain what 'caring' means to you.

✔ What do you think the difference is between a support worker caring for a patient and a nurse caring for a patient?

Questioning the Selectors

The interview is a two-way process and you get an opportunity at the end of the interview to put forward some questions of your own. The two main benefits of asking questions are:

✔ The interviewer gets the impression that you're interested in the university and are motivated to become one of their students.

✔ You get more information to help you decide whether the university is the right one for you.

Do your research about the university, its nursing programme and about the clinical areas that student nurses work in. If the university has specific literature or a website then check the information available there. Having this information beforehand ensures you ask the most appropriate questions.

When writing the questions keep these pointers in mind:

✔ Leave the interviewer with a positive picture of you.

✔ Make clear from your questions that you are interested in being a student at the university.

✔ Ask questions that are meaningful to the interview, and not off topic or covering aspects of the programme already covered in the selection event/interview.

✔ Don't ask questions in a way that may make the interviewer feel you're trying to test her or catch her out over details or specifics.

Here are some questions that make a positive impression:

✔ Can you please explain how supervision is given for help with assignments?

✔ Are there any special or unusual clinical areas that students can attend as part of their learning?

✔ How is the mentoring of students arranged in clinical practice?

✔ Can you please explain how the clinical and academic parts of the programme are managed?

✔ Are there opportunities to get involved with university life such as student ambassadors or nursing unions?

Five questions not to ask your interviewer

When you ask the following questions, the interviewer may make a judgement of you as follows:

✔ 'How much is the bursary and when do I get paid?' In comparison to other university students nursing has a generous bursary support; you don't want to leave the interviewer with the impression you are only applying for the money.

✔ 'Will I have to work weekends and night shifts?' You're expected to work similar shifts as the rest of the nursing team; giving the impression that you want more sociable shift patterns doesn't demonstrate commitment.

✔ 'Can you explain to me how often I have to go into clinical practice?' While you may ask this question because you're eager to work in practice, it can be misconstrued that you'd rather spend more time on campus than working with patients.

✔ 'If I don't like adult nursing is there the opportunity to transfer to mental health nursing?' This question suggests that you don't really understand the different nursing fields and lack commitment to one or the other.

✔ 'Does being "supernumerary" mean I don't have to do "hands-on" care?' Students are expected to be fully involved in nursing care and don't simply observe. Interviewers are looking for candidates willing to participate in all aspects of care.

Prepare your questions in advance and keep a copy with your documents to take on the day. Write five or six questions and practise asking them out loud.

Don't be afraid to take the list of questions into the interview with you and read from your list. You aren't expected to memorise your questions.

Chapter 17

Getting Your Results and Making Decisions

. . . .

. . . .

*I*n some ways the results part of the application process is just as stressful as writing your personal statement or attending an interview. You've no doubt experienced the anxiety of waiting to receive exam results and the turmoil of emotions that you go through before you open the letter and see the results. Waiting for universities to make their decisions on your application is no different, and expect a rollercoaster of emotions as each decision is recorded on your UCAS account.

Hopefully, you receive offers. Alternatively, you may receive rejections that either limit your options or draw your nursing application to a close for that year.

This chapter explores the process of receiving results, both positive and disappointing, and what the different terminology means in relation to your application. I explain the options that you have and how to choose the best strategy for dealing with a variety of results.

Waiting to hear the result of each of your choices can be very frustrating. Contacting individual universities for updates doesn't speed up the decision-making process. Universities inform you through the Track section of the UCAS system on set dates, so be patient.

Handling Successful Offers

Hopefully, your application is successful and you start to receive positive responses from all your choices. Although offers feel great, making decisions that will shape your future course can be a source of anxiety. Read on to put your mind at ease.

Looking at the offers

Your options become clearer as the universities to which you've applied make decisions on each of your choices. Your full options won't become clear for some time because universities have different approaches to making decisions that include:

- ✔ Considering applications as they arrive or immediately after interview, so you receive a decision very quickly.

- ✔ Making a decision on the very good and not so good applications straight away, but keeping the others until all applications have been reviewed.

- ✔ Not making any decisions until after the closing date or after all the interviews have been conducted, so candidates are judged all together.

Chapter 16 covers the interview. If successful at interview, a university makes you an offer in one of two ways:

- ✔ **Unconditional offers:** You meet all the academic requirements, and the university is happy to accept you.

- ✔ **Conditional offers:** The university will offer you a place if you meet certain conditions. These conditions are academic related and usually require you to pass your exams and meet the points or grades.

For both types of offer the university attaches additional conditions to the offer that include a satisfactory Criminal Records Bureau (CRB) and health check (see Chapter 4) and references (see Chapter 13).

Making your decision

As each university makes a decision about your application, this is displayed on your UCAS profile, but you can't act on any of these decisions until all the universities you applied to have responded. This is to stop you from making any rash decisions before you know all your options.

You normally have approximately four to five weeks to reply if all your chosen universities have responded by the end of March. If you apply later in the application cycle then the universities have less time to make their decisions and you have less time to reply. Your reply date shows up in the Track section of the UCAS system (see Chapter 11). Don't worry if the date is different to your friends' dates; this is quite normal.

When reviewing your options:

- ✔ Carefully check the terms of the offer. Some conditions may apply, such as gaining certain grades or specific start dates.

- ✔ Don't panic and accept the first offer that arrives. You have time to think about the choices you have.

- ✔ Make sure you make a decision by the deadline date in UCAS Track. If you don't then the offer will be rejected automatically by UCAS.

- ✔ Keep your correspondence details updated, otherwise you may miss important information. You can do this in Track.

- ✔ Should there be any changes to your circumstances that could affect your results, such as ill health, contact the university straight away. Don't leave it until your results are published.

If you have more than one offer then you choose just one university as your main choice and a second university as your 'insurance'. Remember that:

- ✔ You will be automatically placed in your insurance university if you don't meet the conditions for your first choice.

- ✔ Your insurance choice only accepts you if you meet their conditions, so it is not advisable to pick an insurance university with higher entry requirements than your first choice.

- ✔ You don't have to accept your insurance choice and can enter into clearing if you want.

You can make several decisions based on the amount of choices and offers received:

- ✔ **Firm acceptance:** This is your first and preferred choice from all the offers you have received. You can only have one firm acceptance, and if you accept an unconditional offer then you must decline all the other offers.

- ✔ **Insurance acceptance:** If your firm choice was against a conditional offer you're able to make a second choice. This is a reserve choice and is your backup plan should you not meet the conditions for your firm choice.

Think carefully about your insurance choice. Should the conditions of the offer for the insurance choice be higher than those of your firm choice, it's unlikely you will be accepted by an insurance university if you don't meet the conditions of your first choice.

✔ **Decline:** Once you have made your firm and insurance choices you need to decline all the other offers.

You end up replying with one of four possible combinations:

✔ **Unconditional firm:** You accept an unconditional offer and therefore can't make any other choices

✔ **Conditional firm only:** You make your first choice and either have no other offers to choose from or choose to reject all other offers.

✔ **Conditional firm and conditional insurance:** You make your first choice and select an insurance choice as well; both have conditions attached.

✔ **Conditional firm and unconditional insurance:** Your first choice has conditions attached but your insurance choice doesn't.

If you receive offers that you know you want to accept, then you can make your decision straight away. To do this use Track to withdraw from any outstanding choices.

Be 100 per cent certain that the offer is right for you. Once you withdraw your choices they can't be reversed. Don't rush in and make a rash decision that you later regret. However, don't procrastinate and delay your decision too long. Should UCAS not receive your reply before the set dates, it automatically rejects the offers.

You don't have to accept any offers made and can decline them all. If you do this you may then be eligible to use UCAS Extra and clearing to seek other offers (see Chapter 11 and the later section 'Looking at your options' for more on these paths).

Considering adjustment

If you do exceptionally well in your exams and achieve higher grades than expected, you can reconsider your choice of university. The *Adjustment* system helps those students who would have chosen a different university if they had known they would gain better grades. The system is located in the Track section of your UCAS account.

Helpful hints for choosing your uni

Here are some top tips to help you make a good decision:

✔ Use your evaluation matrix from the open days (see Chapter 9) to remind you of the impression you had of each university. The positive and negative thoughts you had then can influence your decision now.

✔ If you didn't attend an open day and there is still time, make an impromptu visit to the campus to see whether you feel if it's right for you.

✔ Don't let emotion get in the way of making the more sensible decision. Use your instincts and weigh up the pros and cons.

✔ Take advice from someone you trust to give a balanced opinion, but remember that ultimately it is you who makes the decision.

Although Adjustment is a useful option, bear these points in mind:

✔ Universities need to have vacancies in order to consider you.

✔ You have to exceed the condition of your first choice.

✔ You can't use Adjustment if your original offer was unconditional.

✔ You only have five days to consider this option, which may not be long enough to make all the necessary plans to commit to start the programme.

Asking for a deferral

So far you have spent a considerable amount of time and energy focusing on the prospect of going to university. It seems somewhat peculiar to now discuss the possibility of delaying the take up of any offers you've received.

But each year many thousands of students put back the start date of their course, and it is quite common to hear of students taking a 'gap year' before starting their course.

Most universities advertise whether they accept deferred applications. The UCAS application system has a section in which you indicate your wish to defer your place and this is highlighted to the admissions team so they can make the necessary arrangements when calculating student numbers.

If you make a deferred application to a university that doesn't offer deferred places then your application is rejected. Don't lose opportunities with your choices by not checking all the entry criteria.

You may defer in order to:

- ✔ Take a breather between academic study to work, rest or have fun.
- ✔ Travel the world, visit faraway countries and taste alternative cultures.
- ✔ Gain some additional experience and develop your skill base.
- ✔ Have time to prepare all your commitments ready for university.
- ✔ Find work to help manage your finances.

If you didn't request a deferred place on your initial application and subsequently want to delay your start date, then you need to contact the universities directly. You can't retrospectively alter your application through UCAS after it has been sent.

Here are some things to consider when asking for a deferred place:

- ✔ The university doesn't have to grant your request.
- ✔ There is usually a requirement to explain any extenuating circumstances for the request.
- ✔ Because the deferment could mean many months between your interview and start date, you may be asked to attend an informal meeting prior to starting to ensure you still meet professional requirements.
- ✔ New CRB, health checks and references are requested closer to the start date, any changes could impact on you commencing the programme.
- ✔ You are liable for any additional cost such as updating your CRB.
- ✔ Any fees and bursaries will be charged at the rate on commencing the programme, not when making the application. These could be more costly to you.

Sometime universities defer your offer. This can happen when they have a choice of start dates such as September and March and they allocate you the later start. If this is inconvenient, you can ask for reconsideration, but it's at the admissions tutor's discretion.

Changing your mind

Believe it or not, candidates do change their minds after putting themselves through the stress of applying to nursing. The admissions tutor is used to dealing with such requests. The usual reasons for changing your mind include:

✔ Deciding that you've chosen the wrong field of nursing.

✔ Realising that nursing is not the career for you.

✔ Changing personal circumstances that alter your priorities, such as pregnancy.

✔ Becoming financially unable to go to university.

✔ No longer wanting to study at that particular university.

You can manage withdrawal from choices through Track on your UCAS account. The withdrawn choice counts as one of your maximum five choices.

Be certain that you want to withdraw from your choices because once you have made your decision the withdrawal cannot be reversed. Be clear why you're withdrawing, and if you have already been in touch with the admissions team, such as asking for advice or meeting at selection events, then send them a courtesy email. Approach the situation with a mature and professional attitude, especially if you want to be considered by the same university in the future.

If you've accepted an offer but want to withdraw that decision then speak with the university. They can release you from the offer, which allows you to consider other UCAS options that you may have, such as other offers.

Waiting for the course to start

With the offer in the bag this is the time to feel good. You have worked extremely hard and done yourself proud to gain a place at university. But don't rest on your laurels; you've plenty to do between making your choice and starting the programme:

✔ Concentrate on your studies – you still have to make those grades (unless you're lucky enough to have an unconditional offer, but even then, you want to do well). You don't want to drop your guard now and risk losing that place.

✔ Do you need to arrange accommodation? You may have to apply to your university and spend some time sorting contracts and arranging bonds or references.

✔ Have you completed all the requirements for the professional element of the programme? Have you completed your CRB application form and paid the fee? Is there the occupational health check to complete?

✔ If you have a learning need, talk to the university. Most are happy to discuss your needs before you start your course to ensure you have all the support necessary.

✔ Have you completed all the bursary forms and provided the right documents to claim your full financial entitlements?

✔ You may want to start reading around nursing. It's possible to get reading lists in advance so you can start browsing through the books. Alternatively, reading nursing journals is a good way of preparing yourself.

Dealing with Disappointment

No one likes to be disappointed, but unfortunately it's a fact of life that on occasions you fail to achieve your goals . . . on the first attempt at least! How you cope with your disappointment says much about your character and also about your commitment and motivation to become a nurse. Not gaining the offers you had hoped for doesn't need to be the end of your aspirations, and how you react to decisions now can have an impact on your likelihood of gaining a place later.

UCAS informs you of any decisions through Track, and when you have not been successful this is stated in two ways:

✔ **Unsuccessful application:** The university has decided not to offer you a place on its programme. This may be for a number of reasons and can happen before or after an interview. If the university has stated the reason for your rejection, it shows up alongside the decision in your UCAS account.

✔ **Withdrawn:** Universities have the option to withdraw your application from their selection process. The usual reasons for this include not responding to letters or emails or your failure to attend an interview.

Take these initial steps to help you understand why you haven't yet succeeded and make some meaning of your disappointment:

✔ Don't bottle up your disappointment. Talk to family or friends about how you feel.

✔ Understand the context of the disappointment: the competition is tough and not all candidates succeed.

✔ Don't be harsh on yourself. Recognise the good qualities you have and what you still have to offer.

✔ Talk to your school or college tutors who may be able to help you understand the decisions made by the university.

The following sections help you work through the decisions you make next.

Rooting out the reason for the rejection

Your application may be rejected without you having the opportunity to attend an interview or selection event. Candidates are most often unsuccessful at this stage either because no places are available on the course or because the candidates haven't:

✔ Submitted the application by the deadline date.

✔ Met (or are unlikely to meet) academic entry qualifications.

✔ Completed the application form correctly.

✔ Written the personal statement well.

✔ Met eligibility criteria to receive funding of course fees.

Your application may also be rejected after the interview because you:

✔ Failed to produce required documents on the day.

✔ Performed poorly at interview.

✔ Performed well at interview but didn't achieve high enough scores (including numeracy and literacy) to be selected.

After you've had time to think about the results, you may want to find out more as to why you were rejected. To do this you need to contact the admissions team directly. Wherever possible universities try to offer feedback to all unsuccessful candidates. However, it's very much down to the discretion of the admissions team whether this happens and in what format.

It's likely you want feedback at the busiest period of the admissions process, and many other candidates are also asking for feedback too. This often means that the admissions team can't give personalised or lengthy feedback, and the response you receive is either brief or on a standard format with tick boxes identifying the areas of weakness in your application.

Feedback is useful for preparing yourself for other choices or selection events that may be planned within this application cycle. Alternatively, if you want to re-apply in the future, feedback is useful as a guide to improve your chances of success with a new application. Use feedback constructively to:

- ✔ Reflect on what you may have done wrong or not so well.

- ✔ Be honest with yourself about your suitability to nursing.

- ✔ Develop an action plan for improving future applications.

Looking at your options

You have several options to manage any setbacks depending on the number of choices you made and the point you have reached in the application cycle.

Making further choices

If you haven't used all your five choices it is possible to add further choices through your UCAS account. You don't have to make all five choices when first submitting your application, and if you are a little undecided about where to apply, sometimes it's wise to hold back choices until you're more sure of your intentions. Here are some points to consider:

- ✔ You need to pay an additional fee to UCAS to add more choices if you only made one choice originally.

- ✔ Making choices after 15 January limits which universities you can apply to because many use this date as a cutoff point for accepting applications.

- ✔ You can't change your personal statement on UCAS from the one originally submitted. This may not be helpful if you now apply to a different field of nursing.

Using Extra

If you've used all five choices and are not holding any offers then you may be eligible to use Extra. This service allows you to apply for other courses not included in your original five choices. Keep in mind that:

- ✔ Extra is only available between February and July.

- ✔ You can only choose one course at a time.

- ✔ If you accept an offer through Extra, you can't apply elsewhere.

Before making an application through Extra, check the course status on UCAS, which indicates whether places are available. You don't want to make a pointless application.

Using clearing

If by July you have no offers then you can use clearing to apply for courses. Clearing is the process often used after A-level results are published in August whereby students not holding any offers try to find any places that universities still have vacant. Here's how it works:

✔ You approach the universities directly and don't go through UCAS.

✔ You can contact as many universities at the same time as you want.

✔ If a university makes you an offer, you need to put their course details into your UCAS account to enable the university to formalise the offer.

Have your clearing number and your exam results at hand, as the admissions tutors ask for these when speaking with you on the phone.

If you're unable to secure a place through clearing then you need to understand that for this year you've been unsuccessful.

Re-applying

If you're unable to get a place on a nursing course, your initial knee jerk reaction may be to throw in the towel and forget about nursing altogether. Be realistic. If feedback suggested that maybe nursing is not for you, take this as a sign to change career aspirations. It's highly likely you'll be unsuccessful again. But equally if you were a good candidate, but didn't quite make the cut, give serious consideration to the option of re-applying.

It's very common for candidates who are unsuccessful in one year to be successful in the next. Some admissions teams see re-application as a positive feature of your character because it demonstrates commitment and motivation. Don't be embarrassed that you weren't successful on your first attempt.

All the preparatory work from your last application helps make your new application easier. But don't be complacent.

Remember that if you re-apply to the same university they have your previous application form. It's easy to see whether you've just copied your old application or attempted to develop and improve upon your last try.

Don't use your old personal statement; update it. Double-check that entry criteria and selection events haven't changed. And check for any changes to fees and bursaries.

Show your commitment and determination by indicating that you took on board the reason for rejection and worked on any areas of weakness.

Part VI
The Part of Tens

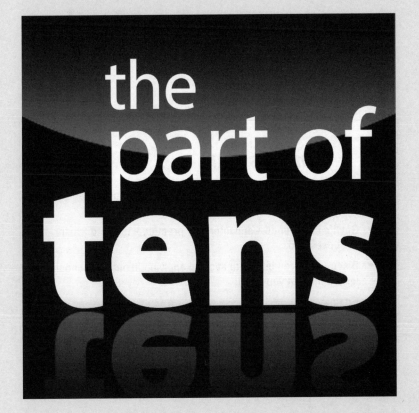

Go to www.dummies.com/extras/getintonursing schooluk for free online bonus content, including a bonus Part of Tens chapter created especially for this book.

In this part . . .

✔ Read tips on planning ahead and getting a strategy in place for your application to nursing school.

✔ Get life experience – and interview practice – to stand you in the best stead.

✔ Discover the ten pitfalls to avoid in applying to nursing school – ignore them at your peril!

✔ Go to www.dummies.com/extras/getintonursing schooluk for online bonus content including an extra Part of Tens chapter: 'Ten Tips for Controlling Stress'.

Chapter 18

Ten Tips for a Successful Application

Throughout the book I offer guidance to help give you the best chance of a successful application. In this chapter, I offer my very best tips – follow these and you're bound to impress an admissions tutor.

Plan Your Time Early

You can't underestimate the amount of time it takes to fully prepare your application to nursing. Few applications are successful when they're rushed at the last moment with little thought or preparation.

 Make yourself a schedule on which you chart things to do and when you'll do them. Doing so helps you manage your preparations smoothly and without stress. Chapter 1 gives you an idea of how long the whole process can take and you can use that as an example to help plan your own timeline.

Develop a Research Strategy

Understanding nursing and healthcare is essential for a successful application. No admissions tutor is going to offer you a place when you don't really know what nursing is or how healthcare works. Just stating the bare facts about nursing isn't sufficient – you need to have a good understanding of what nurses do and, in particular, the role of the nurse for your chosen field.

Research means finding out and investigating nursing, a good start is to use the internet. Type some nursing words, such as 'NHS nursing careers', into a search engine. Read nursing journals for a wealth of useful information. The *Nursing Standard* or the *Nursing Times* are good examples.

Talk to Other Candidates

You're not alone; many thousands of people like yourself all over the UK are considering a nursing degree. They have the same anxieties as you, ask the same questions and undertake the same research. So tap into this rich source of information and find out how others are preparing for university.

Talking to people who are going through the same experiences as you is a good way of gauging that you're on the right track with your preparations. If fellow candidates seem to know more than you then you know you have more investigating to do, but if you find that you're learning little new information then you've probably absorbed as much knowledge as you need.

Many forums and blogs online allow students to share experiences, ask questions and give advice, and some have dedicated sections for nursing students, so the information is specific to your needs.

If you're not sure where to start looking, try The Student Room (www.thestudentroom.co.uk) and search for 'Nursing and Midwifery Forum', where you find over 20,000 different posts.

Gain Expert Advice

Take the effort to contact those who have experience in nursing and applications. They can give you inside knowledge of what to do to perfect your application, and can warn you of pitfalls to avoid and any potential changes to the selection process.

The university prospectus or website gives you the name of the admissions tutor for your chosen field, who'll be happy to advise on specific questions you may have.

If you send a standard email, you receive a standard reply. Personalise the email and address the admissions tutor by name; in this way you're likely to receive a much more informative and individual response.

Create a Good Impression

First impressions count! Don't underestimate the power of the first encounter with the admissions team. You can stand out from the crowd in many ways, but make sure these are positive impressions.

A poorly constructed email asking for information which is freely available on the university website doesn't impress! When visiting universities remember that your suitability for nursing is constantly being assessed; Chapters 9 and 14 give more advice about the selection process.

Remain Motivated

Even the most motivated candidate can feel unmotivated at times. Preparation of your nursing application can take a long time and from conception to acceptance you have many hurdles to clear before you succeed with your ambition. Recognise that you'll have bad times as well as good. Keep focused on your ultimate goal, and plan out small steps to achieve along the way. You're more likely to succeed if you keep motivated, as you're more positive in your attitude towards the application process.

Gain Interview Experience

Often the difference between an offer and a rejection is how you perform at interview. Most candidates score reasonably well at interview but don't *excel* – due to interview nerves rather than not being suitable. Being confident at interview and having the ability to express your thoughts comes only from practice, and a few uncomfortable hours being 'interviewed' by a parent or friend just might get you that offer. For more on preparing for your interview, head to Chapter 16.

Keep in Touch

Once introductions have been made and your application is being considered, make sure that you keep in communication with the admissions team. Don't bombard them with emails each week, wanting an update on progress, but tentatively keep your application in the 'consideration' pile by making sure you reply to any requests promptly, and send a polite email of thanks if you have attended a talk or visit. Remember to let the admissions tutor know if you change your details, such as your address, otherwise you may miss important information.

Get Some Life Experience

Although having some care experience is good, not all universities require it. To develop your interpersonal skills, I recommend gaining some experience working in the community with other people. In doing so you practise your communication and social skills and develop those people skills the admissions tutors look for (for more on people skills, see Chapter 5).

Working with others develops your self-esteem and confidence in how to behave and talk in front of others. These are essential skills for the selection process (see Part V).

Put Your Documents in Order

Each significant event of your life is documented, and you need the documents as proof of your existence and eligibility. Universities only accept original copies, and those which seem to cause problems to replace for candidates are academic, birth or marriage certificates.

If you can't provide the documents the university needs then your application will be rejected. It can take considerable time to replace your certificates if they have been mislaid, so read the advice in Part IV to perfect your application.

Chapter 19

Ten Common Pitfalls to Navigate

· ·

In This Chapter

▶ Ensuring the application is error-free

▶ Following instructions to the letter

▶ Demonstrating people skills and professional behaviour

· ·

*I*n all the years I've been working as an admissions tutor, I've seen many thousands of applications from prospective nursing students. With this experience comes the knowledge that many candidates struggle with their applications because they fail to navigate some common pitfalls.

In this chapter, I outline the reasons that admissions tutors often rejects candidates. Avoid these pitfalls and you increase your chances of success and have a far more comfortable (dare I say enjoyable?) experience of the application process.

Ignoring Entry Criteria

The purpose of entry criteria is to set the minimum standard you must meet for the university to consider you for the programme. These standards are set to ensure that the university chooses the most appropriate students and also that you have the best potential to complete the degree. For nursing, standards are quite detailed because they include both the academic and the professional qualifications that you work towards.

Each university advertises what it expects to see in your application. Ignoring this information is only going to result in an unsuccessful decision. So, if the university asks for 360 UCAS points and you only have 280 points, you're going to get a straight rejection. Likewise if the criteria include A-level biology and you only have a GCSE then expect your application to be refused.

Also review your eligibility for NHS finances. If you don't meet the criteria to receive funding, you're better off delaying your application until you're eligible than submitting an application that has no chance of success.

If you don't quite meet the entry criteria, don't send off your application in the hope the admissions tutor will look kindly on you. Contact the tutor beforehand and discuss your chances to save wasting a choice.

Assessing entry criteria is very straightforward: either you have the qualifications or you haven't. Don't expect the admissions tutor to second-guess which qualifications you have or how you meet the entry criteria. You need to explain the facts clearly on your form.

Leaving Errors in Your Application Form

The information you provide on your application form is all the admissions tutor has to make an initial assessment of your suitability. In all probability the tutor will review your form alongside hundreds of others, so your form needs something special to get the tutor's attention. Make sure that 'something' isn't special for the wrong reasons! Mistakes and omissions give the admissions tutor an easy reason to reject your application.

Here are key areas to focus on:

- ✔ **Writing quality:** Make sure you've written accurately and well. Complete all the text in a word-processed document on your computer, use the spell check and proofread thoroughly, then cut and paste into your UCAS account. See Chapter 12 for more details on perfecting your writing.

- ✔ **References:** They can make a difference. College and school tutors are very good at writing references, but if you're using someone else as your referee, that person may not understand the UCAS system. Speak with the referee and clearly explain the sort of information he needs to include. Flick to Chapter 13 for the lowdown on references.

- ✔ **Qualifications:** The admissions tutors need to know that you have the right qualifications. If you input your qualifications incorrectly, they don't always show up on your application form. Don't expect the admissions tutor to guess or ask for more information.

Applying to Multiple Nursing Fields

Competition for each of the nursing fields is very high and each admissions tutor is looking for the candidate that demonstrates the greatest potential. Each field has its own characteristics and career pathways that are distinctly different to those of other fields. The admissions tutor often takes the view that you need to have a clear appreciation of the field of nursing to which you apply.

 Some universities don't consider applications to numerous fields. So if you're contemplating applying to several fields at the same university, seek advice first so your application isn't rejected or delayed. You risk the admissions tutor judging you as not committed to a particular field.

 A common pitfall is to apply to midwifery first but be unsuccessful and so apply to either child or adult nursing. Some candidates believe that it's easy to undertake extra training to become a midwife at a later date. These applications have a high failure rate as the admissions tutor knows your heart lies with midwifery and your personal statement supports midwifery not nursing. (Chapter 12 has more advice on writing your personal statement.)

Failing to Keep Contact Details Up-to-date

When completing your UCAS application form you have the opportunity to give a couple of different ways for universities to communicate with you – usually, postal address, email and telephone.

Keep these details up to date so that both UCAS and universities can correspond with you about your application. Many universities contact you directly, and not all information about progress is recorded on your UCAS account, so a change of details can lead to you missing vital information with detrimental results.

 Double-check the settings on your email account because you may find that it automatically directs certain emails into the junk folder. This is a common reason for candidates missing important information.

Don't expect universities to take a lenient view on your missed opportunities due to incorrect details. It's your responsibility to keep your records up-to-date.

Being Complacent about the Competition

It still surprises me how many candidates don't appreciate the challenges of applying for nursing. Sufficient information is given at open days and school and college events to make you aware that nursing is a very competitive degree programme, so you've got to really work hard to stand out in your application.

Not understanding the level of competition usually means that you aren't as prepared for the selection process as many of your competitors. It becomes clear very quickly by reading application forms and talking to candidates which ones have done their research and which ones haven't.

The majority of candidates research and prepare their application to a very high standard. If you don't appreciate this and don't put a great deal of effort into your application, don't expect to be successful.

Confusing Your Experiences

Gaining care experience (see Chapter 6) is an excellent way to prove that nursing is right for you, and it also demonstrates to the admissions tutor that you're up to the challenge. However care experience can be a double-edged sword and many candidates trip themselves up trying to explain how their experiences support their understanding of nursing.

Experience of hands-on care is often a good way to prepare for nursing and it helps you to understand the practicalities of nursing practice. But it is too easy to concentrate on what *you* have gained from the experience, what *you* liked about caring and how the experience helped *you* decide why you want to be a nurse, rather than explaining what you have to offer the *nursing profession*.

Admissions tutors know what students get from nursing; after all they are nurses themselves. What they want to know is what you bring to nursing. You need to turn your experiences on their head and not think what you take from nursing, but what you can give to your patients.

Ignoring Instructions and Requests

Even if you think you've already answered all of his queries, if an admissions tutor asks for more information or gives you further instructions, don't ignore them.

In the course of assessing your application the university requires many different forms and documents, ranging from your original academic transcripts to character references. Some candidates fail to respond promptly or, in some cases, at all. The university has deadlines to meet and is likely to then reject your application.

 Admissions tutors have many candidates waiting in the wings to take up any places that become available. They have no qualms about rejecting your application if you don't follow instructions, because they know there are other candidates who will.

Being Too Creative

In the desire to be successful, it's quite understandable that you feel compelled to portray yourself in the best possible light to the admissions team. Illustrating your skills and qualities in your personal statement and at interview in a way that suggests you make the ideal student is quite acceptable.

The difficulty is finding the fine line between representing your skills and abilities in an optimistic way and suggesting that you have qualities that you don't. The information you provide in your personal statement and at interview can be challenged and often requires corroboration through other sources such as references. Be sure you can substantiate any claims you make. For more on personal statements and interviews, visit Chapters 12, 14 and 16.

Demonstrating Poor Communication and Social Skills

It's a requirement that you have some face-to-face contact with the admissions team before they make you an offer. The reason for this is to review your attitude and behaviour and check your suitability to work with vulnerable members of the public.

Many candidates are unsuccessful because they can't talk freely and build a rapport with other candidates and interviewers at selection events. These candidates don't appreciate the skills that are being assessed. Nursing isn't just about academia, and having excellent qualifications doesn't automatically make you a strong candidate. Nurses use a range of communication and social skills to interact with patients, and these are given equal consideration when decisions are made.

Put as much effort into developing your communication and social skills as you do in writing your personal statement and preparing for your interview.

Chapter 5 helps you understand the people skills required, and Part V helps you through selection days.

Lacking Integrity

It still surprises me how many candidates are unable to make the connection between the professional behaviour expected of nursing students and their own behaviour during the selection process.

Offers are withdrawn on professional grounds if your good character is brought into question.

Making excuses for errors, passing the blame onto others or plagiarising personal statements are just some examples of behaviour that doesn't support your application. Approach your application with the same professional attitude that you understand is expected of you once you're a student nurse.

Index

• R •

• S •

About the Author

Andrew Evered, RN, MSc (Econ), PCGE came to nursing after a few years in the finance industry and qualified as an Adult Registered Nurse in 1988. Specialising in medical nursing, Andrew spent many years working as a staff nurse in a general hospital caring for patients with respiratory and cardiac conditions. After several years consolidating his nursing experience, Andrew moved into a senior nurse role advising and supporting nurses with regards to their education and professional practice.

With an interest in teaching and recruitment, Andrew undertook further study, gaining qualifications in research, management and teaching.

Andrew's professional interests are in selection and recruitment and he undertook research into nurse retention for national government and helped develop recruitment strategies for his local health board.

Andrew is currently a senior lecturer at Swansea University teaching both pre-and post-registration nursing students. He is also a personal tutor for pre-registration students and takes an active role in their professional and pastoral development.

Andrew is the lead admissions tutor for pre-registration nursing programmes and has extensive knowledge in the selection of nursing students.

Publisher's Acknowledgments

We're proud of this book; please send us your comments at http://dummies.cust help.com. For other comments, please contact our Customer Care Department within the U.S. at 877-762-2974, outside the U.S. at (001) 317-572-3993, or fax 317-572-4002.

Some of the people who helped bring this book to market include the following:

Acquisitions, Editorial, and Vertical Websites

Commissioning Editor: Mike Baker

Project Editor: Rachael Chilvers

Assistant Editor: Ben Kemble

Development Editor: Charlie Wilson

Technical Editor: Tina Attoe, Admissions Tutor, School of Nursing and Midwifery, University of Brighton

Proofreader: James Harrison

Production Manager: Daniel Mersey

Publisher: Miles Kendall

Cover Photo: © Andrew Hill / iStockphoto

Composition Services

Senior Project Coordinator: Kristie Rees

Layout and Graphics: Amy Hassos, Kathie Rickard

Indexer: Potomoc Indexing, LLC

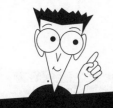

FOR DUMMIES®

Making Everything Easier!™

UK editions

BUSINESS

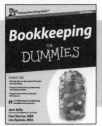

Bookkeeping For Dummies
978-1-118-34689-1

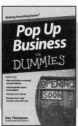

Pop Up Business For Dummies
978-1-118-44349-1

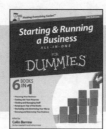

Starting & Running a Business All-in-One For Dummies
978-1-119-97527-4

MUSIC

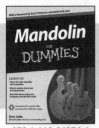

Mandolin For Dummies
978-1-119-94276-4

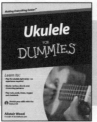

Ukulele For Dummies
978-0-470-97799-6

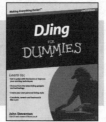

DJing For Dummies
978-0-470-66372-1

HOBBIES

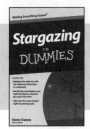

Stargazing For Dummies
978-1-118-41156-8

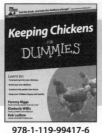

Keeping Chickens For Dummies
978-1-119-99417-6

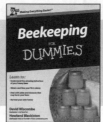

Beekeeping For Dummies
978-1-119-97250-1

Asperger's Syndrome For Dummies
978-0-470-66087-4

Basic Maths For Dummies
978-1-119-97452-9

Body Language For Dummies,
2nd Edition
978-1-119-95351-7

Boosting Self-Esteem For Dummies
978-0-470-74193-1

Business Continuity For Dummies
978-1-118-32683-1

Cricket For Dummies
978-0-470-03454-5

Diabetes For Dummies, 3rd Edition
978-0-470-97711-8

eBay For Dummies, 3rd Edition
978-1-119-94122-4

English Grammar For Dummies
978-0-470-05752-0

Flirting For Dummies
978-0-470-74259-4

IBS For Dummies
978-0-470-51737-6

ITIL For Dummies
978-1-119-95013-4

Management For Dummies,
2nd Edition
978-0-470-97769-9

Managing Anxiety with CBT
For Dummies
978-1-118-36606-6

Neuro-linguistic Programming
For Dummies,
2nd Edition
978-0-470-66543-5

Nutrition For Dummies,
2nd Edition
978-0-470-97276-2

Organic Gardening For Dummies
978-1-119-97706-3

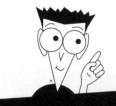

FOR **DUMMIES®**

Making Everything Easier!™

UK editions

SELF-HELP

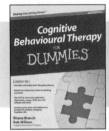

Cognitive Behavioural Therapy For Dummies
978-0-470-66541-1

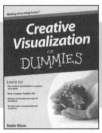

Creative Visualization For Dummies
978-1-119-99264-6

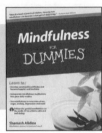

Mindfulness For Dummies
978-0-470-66086-7

LANGUAGES

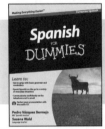

Spanish For Dummies
978-0-470-68815-1

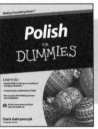

Polish For Dummies
978-1-119-97959-3

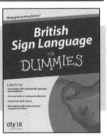

British Sign Language For Dummies
978-0-470-69477-0

HISTORY

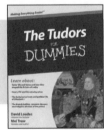

The Tudors For Dummies
978-0-470-68792-5

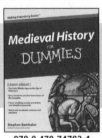

Medieval History For Dummies
978-0-470-74783-4

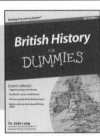

British History For Dummies
978-0-470-97819-1

Origami Kit For Dummies
978-0-470-75857-1

Overcoming Depression
For Dummies
978-0-470-69430-5

Positive Psychology For Dummies
978-0-470-72136-0

PRINCE2 For Dummies,
2009 Edition
978-0-470-71025-8

Project Management For Dummies
978-0-470-71119-4

Psychology Statistics For Dummies
978-1-119-95287-9

Psychometric Tests For Dummies
978-0-470-75366-8

Renting Out Your Property
For Dummies, 3rd Edition
978-1-119-97640-0

Rugby Union For Dummies,
3rd Edition
978-1-119-99092-5

Sage One For Dummies
978-1-119-95236-7

Self-Hypnosis For Dummies
978-0-470-66073-7

Storing and Preserving Garden
Produce For Dummies
978-1-119-95156-8

Teaching English as a Foreign
Language For Dummies
978-0-470-74576-2

Time Management For Dummies
978-0-470-77765-7

Training Your Brain For Dummies
978-0-470-97449-0

Voice and Speaking Skills
For Dummies
978-1-119-94512-3

Work-Life Balance For Dummies
978-0-470-71380-8

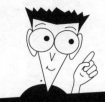

FOR DUMMIES®

Making Everything Easier!™

COMPUTER BASICS

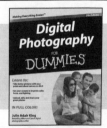

978-1-118-11533-6

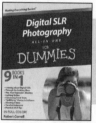

978-0-470-61454-9

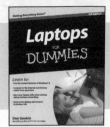

978-0-470-49743-2

DIGITAL PHOTOGRAPHY

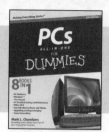

978-1-118-09203-3

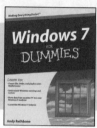

978-0-470-76878-5

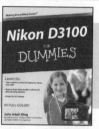

978-1-118-00472-2

SCIENCE AND MATHS

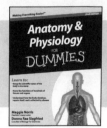

978-0-470-92326-9

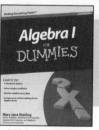

978-0-470-55964-2

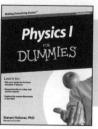

978-0-470-90324-7

Art For Dummies
978-0-7645-5104-8

**Computers For Seniors
For Dummies, 3rd Edition**
978-1-118-11553-4

Criminology For Dummies
978-0-470-39696-4

**Currency Trading For Dummies,
2nd Edition**
978-0-470-01851-4

Drawing For Dummies, 2nd Edition
978-0-470-61842-4

Forensics For Dummies
978-0-7645-5580-0

French For Dummies, 2nd Edition
978-1-118-00464-7

Guitar For Dummies, 2nd Edition
978-0-7645-9904-0

Hinduism For Dummies
978-0-470-87858-3

Index Investing For Dummies
978-0-470-29406-2

Islamic Finance For Dummies
978-0-470-43069-9

Knitting For Dummies, 2nd Edition
978-0-470-28747-7

**Music Theory For Dummies,
2nd Edition**
978-1-118-09550-8

Office 2010 For Dummies
978-0-470-48998-7

Piano For Dummies, 2nd Edition
978-0-470-49644-2

Photoshop CS6 For Dummies
978-1-118-17457-9

Schizophrenia For Dummies
978-0-470-25927-6

**WordPress For Dummies,
5th Edition**
978-1-118-38318-6

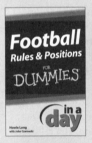
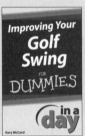
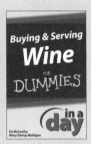
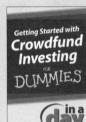
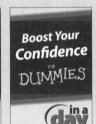
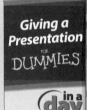
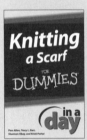
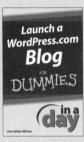
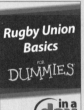
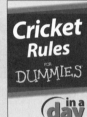
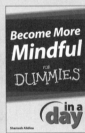
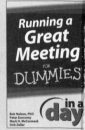
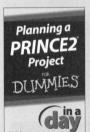
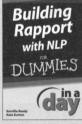
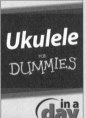
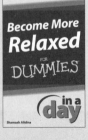